T0368392

Communications
in Computer and Information Science   **2458**

Series Editors

Gang Li ⓘ, *School of Information Technology, Deakin University, Burwood, VIC, Australia*
Joaquim Filipe ⓘ, *Polytechnic Institute of Setúbal, Setúbal, Portugal*
Zhiwei Xu, *Chinese Academy of Sciences, Beijing, China*

Rationale
The CCIS series is devoted to the publication of proceedings of computer science conferences. Its aim is to efficiently disseminate original research results in informatics in printed and electronic form. While the focus is on publication of peer-reviewed full papers presenting mature work, inclusion of reviewed short papers reporting on work in progress is welcome, too. Besides globally relevant meetings with internationally representative program committees guaranteeing a strict peer-reviewing and paper selection process, conferences run by societies or of high regional or national relevance are also considered for publication.

Topics
The topical scope of CCIS spans the entire spectrum of informatics ranging from foundational topics in the theory of computing to information and communications science and technology and a broad variety of interdisciplinary application fields.

Information for Volume Editors and Authors
Publication in CCIS is free of charge. No royalties are paid, however, we offer registered conference participants temporary free access to the online version of the conference proceedings on SpringerLink (http://link.springer.com) by means of an http referrer from the conference website and/or a number of complimentary printed copies, as specified in the official acceptance email of the event.

CCIS proceedings can be published in time for distribution at conferences or as postproceedings, and delivered in the form of printed books and/or electronically as USBs and/or e-content licenses for accessing proceedings at SpringerLink. Furthermore, CCIS proceedings are included in the CCIS electronic book series hosted in the SpringerLink digital library at http://link.springer.com/bookseries/7899. Conferences publishing in CCIS are allowed to use Online Conference Service (OCS) for managing the whole proceedings lifecycle (from submission and reviewing to preparing for publication) free of charge.

Publication process
The language of publication is exclusively English. Authors publishing in CCIS have to sign the Springer CCIS copyright transfer form, however, they are free to use their material published in CCIS for substantially changed, more elaborate subsequent publications elsewhere. For the preparation of the camera-ready papers/files, authors have to strictly adhere to the Springer CCIS Authors' Instructions and are strongly encouraged to use the CCIS LaTeX style files or templates.

Abstracting/Indexing
CCIS is abstracted/indexed in DBLP, Google Scholar, EI-Compendex, Mathematical Reviews, SCImago, Scopus. CCIS volumes are also submitted for the inclusion in ISI Proceedings.

How to start
To start the evaluation of your proposal for inclusion in the CCIS series, please send an e-mail to ccis@springer.com

Yanchun Zhang · Qingcai Chen · Hongfei Lin ·
Lei Liu · Xiangwen Liao · Buzhou Tang ·
Tianyong Hao · Zhengxing Huang · Jianbo Lei ·
Zuofeng Li · Hui Zong
Editors

Health Information Processing

Evaluation Track Papers

10th China Health Information Processing Conference, CHIP 2024
Fuzhou, China, November 15–17, 2024
Proceedings

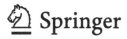 Springer

Editors
Yanchun Zhang
Zhejiang Normal University
Jinhua, China

Hongfei Lin ⓘ
Dalian University of Technology
Dalian, China

Xiangwen Liao
Fuzhou University
Fuzhou, China

Tianyong Hao ⓘ
South China Normal University
Guangzhou, China

Jianbo Lei ⓘ
Medical Informatics Center of Peking
University
Beijing, China

Hui Zong ⓘ
West China Hospital of Sichuan University
Chengdu, China

Qingcai Chen ⓘ
Harbin Institute of Technology
Shenzhen, China

Lei Liu
Fudan University
Shanghai, China

Buzhou Tang ⓘ
Harbin Institute of Technology
Shenzhen, China

Zhengxing Huang
Zhejiang University
Hangzhou, China

Zuofeng Li ⓘ
Takeda Co. Ltd
Shanghai, China

ISSN 1865-0929   ISSN 1865-0937 (electronic)
Communications in Computer and Information Science
ISBN 978-981-96-4297-7   ISBN 978-981-96-4298-4 (eBook)
https://doi.org/10.1007/978-981-96-4298-4

© The Editor(s) (if applicable) and The Author(s), under exclusive license
to Springer Nature Singapore Pte Ltd. 2025

This work is subject to copyright. All rights are solely and exclusively licensed by the Publisher, whether
the whole or part of the material is concerned, specifically the rights of translation, reprinting, reuse of
illustrations, recitation, broadcasting, reproduction on microfilms or in any other physical way, and transmission
or information storage and retrieval, electronic adaptation, computer software, or by similar or dissimilar
methodology now known or hereafter developed.
The use of general descriptive names, registered names, trademarks, service marks, etc. in this publication
does not imply, even in the absence of a specific statement, that such names are exempt from the relevant
protective laws and regulations and therefore free for general use.
The publisher, the authors and the editors are safe to assume that the advice and information in this book
are believed to be true and accurate at the date of publication. Neither the publisher nor the authors or the
editors give a warranty, expressed or implied, with respect to the material contained herein or for any errors
or omissions that may have been made. The publisher remains neutral with regard to jurisdictional claims in
published maps and institutional affiliations.

This Springer imprint is published by the registered company Springer Nature Singapore Pte Ltd.
The registered company address is: 152 Beach Road, #21-01/04 Gateway East, Singapore 189721, Singapore

If disposing of this product, please recycle the paper.

Preface

Health information processing and applications is one of the essential fields in data-driven life health and clinical medicine and it has been highly active in recent decades. The China Health Information Processing Conference (CHIP) is an annual conference held by the Medical Health and Biological Information Processing Committee of the Chinese Information Processing Society (CIPS) of China, with the theme of "large models and smart healthcare". CHIP is one of the leading conferences in the field of health information processing in China and turned into an international event in 2022. It is also an important platform for researchers and practitioners from academia, business and government departments around the world to share ideas and further promote research and applications in this field. CHIP 2024 was organized by Fuzhou University and the proceedings were published by Springer. CHIP 2024 was held offline, whereby people could connect face-to-face with keynote speeches and presentations.

The CHIP 2024 Evaluation Track released 3 shared tasks, including Syndrome Differentiation Thought in Traditional Chinese Medicine, Lymphoma Information Extraction and Automatic Coding, and Typical Case Diagnosis Consistency. Hundreds of teams from both academia and industry engaged in these shared tasks. Out of these participants, 14 top-performing teams were chosen to submit algorithm papers. Additionally, the organizers of the shared tasks also submitted 5 papers detailing dataset descriptions and task overviews. The 19 papers were selected for publication in this volume after a thorough single-blind peer review process in which each submission received two reviews, and rigorous revisions.

The authors of each paper in this volume reported their novel results of computing methods or applications. The volume cannot cover all aspects of Medical Health and Biological Information Processing but may still inspire insightful thoughts for the readers. We hope that more secrets of Health Information Processing will be unveiled, and that academics will drive more practical developments and solutions.

November 2024

Yanchun Zhang
Qingcai Chen
Hongfei Lin
Lei Liu
Xiangwen Liao
Buzhou Tang
Tianyong Hao
Zhengxing Huang
Jianbo Lei
Zuofeng Li
Hui Zong

Organization

Honorary Chairs

Yanchun Zhang   Zhejiang Normal University, China
Qingcai Chen   Harbin Institute of Technology (Shenzhen), China

General Co-chairs

Hongfei Lin   Dalian University of Technology, China
Lei Liu   Fudan University, China
Xiangwen Liao   Fuzhou University, China

Program Co-chairs

Buzhou Tang   Harbin Institute of Technology (Shenzhen) & Pengcheng Laboratory, China
Yanshan Wang   University of Pittsburgh, USA
Maggie Haitian Wang   Chinese University of Hong Kong, China

Young Scientists Forum Co-chairs

Zhengxing Huang   Zhejiang University, China
Yonghui Wu   University of Florida, USA

Publication Co-chairs

Tianyong Hao   South China Normal University, China
Xinyu He   Liaoning Normal University, China
Wenpeng Lu   Qilu University of Technology, China
Zhichang Zhang   Northwest Normal University, China
Ling Luo   Dalian University of Technology, China
Lu Xiang   Institute of Automation, Chinese Academy of Sciences, China
Yongxian Wu   South China University of Technology, China

Jiao Li   Institute of Medical Information, Chinese
                                 Academy of Medical Sciences, China
Yongjun Zhu   Yonsei University, South Korea

Forum Co-chairs

Zhengxing Huang   Zhejiang University, China
Jun Yan   Yidu Cloud (Beijing) Technology Co., Ltd. China
Haofen Wang   Tongji University, China
Ming Feng   Peking Union Medical College Hospital, China
Zhumin Chen   Shandong University, China
Yi Zhou   Sun Yat-sen University, China
Sendong Zhao   Harbin Institute of Technology, China

Evaluation Co-chairs

Zuofeng Li   Takeda China, China
Jianbo Lei   Medical Informatics Center of Peking University,
                                 China
Hui Zong   West China Hospital, Sichuan University, China

Publicity Co-chairs

Lishuang Li   Dalian University of Technology, China
Yinghui Jin   Zhongnan Hospital of Wuhan University, China
Ping Song   Children's Hospital Affiliated to Chongqing
                                 Medical University, China

Sponsor Co-chairs

Siwei Yu   Guizhou Medical University, China
Yi Zhou   Sun Yat-sen University, China
Buyue Qian   Chaoyang Hospital Affiliated to Capital Medical
                                 University, China
Yonghui Wu   University of Florida, USA

Web Chair

Kunli Zhang   Zhengzhou University, China

Program Committee

Wenping Guo   Taizhou University, China
Hongmin Cai   South China University of Technology, China
Chao Che   Dalian University, China
Mosha Chen   Alibaba, China
Qingcai Chen   Harbin Institute of Technology (Shenzhen), China
Xi Chen   Tencent Technology Co., Ltd., China
Yang Chen   Yidu Cloud (Beijing) Technology Co., Ltd., China
Zhumin Chen   Shandong University, China
Ming Cheng   Zhengzhou University, China
Ruoyao Ding   Guangdong University of Foreign Studies, China
Bin Dong   Ricoh Software Research Center (Beijing) Co.,
                                        Ltd., China
Guohong Fu   Soochow University, China
Yan Gao   Central South University, China
Tianyong Hao   South China Normal University, China
Shizhu He   Institute of Automation, Chinese Academy of
                                        Sciences, China
Zengyou He   Dalian University of Technology, China
Na Hong   Digital China Medical Technology Co., Ltd.,
                                        China
Li Hou   Institute of Medical Information, Chinese
                                        Academy of Medical Sciences, China
Yong Hu   Jinan University, China
Baotian Hu   Harbin University of Technology (Shenzhen),
                                        China
Guimin Huang   Guilin University of Electronic Science and
                                        Technology, China
Zhenghang Huang   Zhejiang University, China
Zhiwei Huang   Southwest Medical University, China
Bo Jin   Dalian University of Technology, China
Xiaoyu Kang   Southwest Medical University, China

Jianbo Lei	Peking University, China
Haomin Li	Children's Hospital of Zhejiang University Medical College, China
Jiao Li	Institute of Medical Information, Chinese Academy of Medical Sciences, China
Jinghua Li	Chinese Academy of Traditional Chinese Medicine, China
Lishuang Li	Dalian University of Technology, China
Linfeng Li	Yidu Cloud (Beijing) Technology Co., Ltd., China
Ru Li	Shanxi University, China
Runzhi Li	Zhengzhou University, China
Shasha Li	National University of Defense Technology, China
Xing Li	Beijing Shenzhengyao Technology Co., Ltd., China
Xin Li	Zhongkang Physical Examination Technology Co., Ltd., China
Yuxi Li	Peking University First Hospital, China
Zuofeng Li	Takeda China, China
Xiangwen Liao	Fuzhou University, China
Hao Lin	University of Electronic Science and Technology, China
Hongfei Lin	Dalian University of Technology, China
Bangtao Liu	Southwest Medical University, China
Song Liu	Qilu University of Technology, China
Lei Liu	Fudan University, China
Shengping Liu	Unisound Co., Ltd., China
Xiaoming Liu	Zhongyuan University of Technology, China
Guan Luo	Institute of Automation, Chinese Academy of Sciences, China
Lingyun Luo	Nanhua University, China
Yamei Luo	Southwest Medical University, China
Hui Lv	Shanghai Jiao Tong University, China
Xudong Lv	Zhejiang University, China
Yao Meng	Lenovo Research Institute, China
Qingliang Miao	Suzhou Aispeech Information Technology Co., Ltd., China
Weihua Peng	Baidu Co., Ltd., China
Buyue Qian	Xi'an Jiaotong University, China
Longhua Qian	Suzhou University, China
Tong Ruan	East China University of Technology, China
Ying Shen	South China University of Technology, China

Xiaofeng Song	Nanjing University of Aeronautics and Astronautics, China
Chengjie Sun	Harbin University of Technology, China
Chuanji Tan	Alibaba Dharma Hall, China
Hongye Tan	Shanxi University, China
Jingyu Tan	Shenzhen Xinkaiyuan Information Technology Development Co., Ltd., China
Binhua Tang	Hehai University, China
Buzhou Tang	Harbin Institute of Technology, Shenzhen, China
Jintao Tang	National Defense University of the People's Liberation Army, China
Qian Tao	South China University of Technology, China
Fei Teng	Southwest Jiaotong University, China
Shengwei Tian	Xinjiang University, China
Dong Wang	Southern Medical University, China
Haitian Wang	Chinese University of Hong Kong, China
Haofen Wang	Tongji University, China
Xiaolei Wang	Hong Kong Institute of Sustainable Development Education, China
Haolin Wang	Chongqing Medical University, China
Yehan Wang	Unisound Intelligent Technology, China
Zhenyu Wang	South China Institute of Technology Software, China
Zhongmin Wang	Jiangsu Provincial People's Hospital, China
Leyi Wei	Shandong University, China
Heng Weng	Guangdong Hospital of Traditional Chinese Medicine, China
Gang Wu	Beijing Knowledge Atlas Technology Co., Ltd., China
Xian Wu	Tencent Technology (Beijing) Co., Ltd., China
Jingbo Xia	Huazhong Agricultural University, China
Lu Xiang	Institute of Automation, Chinese Academy of Sciences, China
Yang Xiang	Pengcheng Laboratory, China
Lei Xu	Shenzhen Polytechnic, China
Liang Xu	Ping An Technology (Shenzhen) Co., Ltd., China
Yan Xu	Beihang University, Microsoft Research Asia, China
Jun Yan	Yidu Cloud (Beijing) Technology Co., Ltd., China
Cheng Yang	Institute of Automation, Chinese Academy of Sciences, China
Hai Yang	East China University of Technology, China
Meijie Yang	Chongqing Medical University, China

Muyun Yang	Harbin University of Technology, China
Zhihao Yang	Dalian University of Technology, China
Hui Ye	Guangzhou University of Traditional Chinese Medicine, China
Dehui Yin	Southwest Medical University, China
Qing Yu	Xinjiang University, China
Liang Yu	Xi'an University of Electronic Science and Technology, China
Siwei Yu	Guizhou Provincial People's Hospital, China
Hongying Zan	Zhengzhou University, China
Hao Zhang	Jilin University, China
Kunli Zhang	Zhengzhou University, China
Weide Zhang	Zhongshan Hospital Affiliated to Fudan University, China
Xiaoyan Zhang	Tongji University, China
Yaoyun Zhang	Alibaba, China
Yijia Zhang	Dalian University of Technology, China
Yuanzhe Zhang	Institute of Automation, Chinese Academy of Sciences, China
Zhichang Zhang	Northwest Normal University, China
Qiuye Zhao	Beijing Big Data Research Institute, China
Sendong Zhao	Harbin Institute of Technology, China
Tiejun Zhao	Harbin Institute of Technology, China
Deyu Zhou	Southeast University, China
Fengfeng Zhou	Jilin University, China
Guangyou Zhou	Central China Normal University, China
Yi Zhou	Sun Yat-sen University, China
Conghui Zhu	Harbin Institute of Technology, China
Shanfeng Zhu	Fudan University, China
Yu Zhu	Sunshine Life Insurance Co., Ltd., China
Quan Zou	University of Electronic Science and Technology, China
Xi Chen	University of Electronic Science and Technology, China
Yansheng Li	Mediway Technology Co., Ltd., China
Daojing He	Harbin Institute of Technology, Shenzhen, China
Yupeng Liu	Harbin University of Science and Technology, China
Xinzhi Sun	First Affiliated Hospital of Zhengzhou University, China
Chuanchao Du	Third People's Hospital of Henan Province, China
Xien Liu	Beijing Huijizhiyi Technology Co., Ltd., China
Shan Nan	Hainan University, China

Xinyu He	Liaoning Normal University, China
Qianqian He	Chongqing Medical University, China
Xing Liu	Third Xiangya Hospital of Central South University, China
Jiayin Wang	Xi'an Jiaotong University, China
Ying Xu	Xi'an Jiaotong University, China
Xin Lai	Xi'an Jiaotong University, China

Contents

Syndrome Differentiation Thought in Traditional Chinese Medicine

Overview of the Evaluation Task for Syndrome Differentiation Thought in Traditional Chinese Medicine in CHIP 2024

Meng Hao[1], Keyu Yao[1], Yuyan Huang[2], Lele Yang[1], Suyuan Peng[1], Zhe Wang[3,4,5(✉)], and Yan Zhu[1(✉)]

[1] Institute of Information on Traditional Chinese Medicine, China Academy of Chinese Medical Sciences, Beijing 100700, China
zhuyan166@126.com

[2] Institute of Basic Theory for Chinese Medicine, China Academy of Chinese Medical Sciences, Beijing 100700, China

[3] Institute of Basic Medical Sciences, Chinese Academy of Medical Sciences, Beijing 100005, China

[4] School of Basic Medicine, Peking Union Medical College, Beijing 100005, China

[5] Institute for Medical Informatics, Statistics and Epidemiology, University of Leipzig, 04103 Leipzig, Germany

Abstract. The evaluation task for syndrome differentiation thought of traditional Chinese medicine (TCM) is a complex and important research task. However, this task presents many challenges due to the complex and specialized nature of TCM texts, as well as the necessity of incorporating extensive expertise for in-depth reasoning and analysis. To address these challenges, we have developed a manually curated and reviewed high-quality TCM syndrome differentiation thought evaluation dataset. This dataset aims to provide a standardized, highly credible, and quantifiable benchmark for assessing the reasoning capabilities of large language models (LLMs) in the field of TCM. It contains 300 TCM medical records, which have been manually cleaned and annotated to ensure the rigor and applicability of the data. Furthermore, the dataset was employed in the evaluation task for syndrome differentiation thought of TCM (http://cips-chip.org.cn/2024/eval1) in CHIP-2024. This task consists of four sub-tasks: clinical information extraction, TCM pathogenesis reasoning, TCM syndrome reasoning, and explanatory summary. In conclusion, this paper reviews and analyzes the methods and the results of the participating teams.

Keywords: large language models · syndrome differentiation thought of traditional Chinese medicine · medical natural language processing · complex scene reasoning

1 Introduction

In recent years, large language models (LLMs) have shown significant potential in the biomedical field. For example, Singhal et al. [1] verified that LLMs have achieved better scores in the MultiMedQA. Additionally, Cui et al. [2] introduced the scGPT for

© The Author(s), under exclusive license to Springer Nature Singapore Pte Ltd. 2025
Y. Zhang et al. (Eds.): CHIP 2024, CCIS 2458, pp. 3–9, 2025.
https://doi.org/10.1007/978-981-96-4298-4_1

the single-cell multi-omics tasks. Moreover, LLMs have been applied in various areas, including hospital discharge summaries [3], accurate differential diagnosis(DDx) [4, 5], medical image analysis [6], medical writing [7]. Furthermore, Google has developed a series of models based on PaLM models for the medical domain, such as Med-PaLM and Med-PaLM2 [1, 8]. Cheng et al. have developed GatorTronGPT [9] for clinical report generation. In the field of traditional Chinese medicine, TCM-GPT [10] supports TCM examination and diagnostic tasks. As these advancements continue of LLMs in the medical domain, a new challenge has emerged concerning the scientific, effective, and standardized evaluation of LLMs.

Currently, several excellent evaluation benchmarks are available, such as the MedQA dataset, which comprises questions from the questions from the U.S. Medical Licensing Examination [11], the MedMCQA dataset, featuring questions from the Indian Medical Entrance Examination [12], and the Qibo-benchmark constructed from high-quality training corpus data in TCM [13]. However, these benchmarks primarily focus on Question-Answer (QA) tasks. And syndrome differentiation thought is a complex task, it not only requires integration of TCM theories, but also demands the incorporation of clinical experiences, Consequently, it necessitates a more comprehensive and holistic evaluation framework.

To address this issue, we systematically summarized the process of TCM syndrome differentiation thought based on existing research foundations. We refined the key steps involved in the evidence-recognition thinking chain: identification and extraction, pathogenesis reasoning, syndrome reasoning, and explanatory summary. Four subtasks were designed to evaluate these key steps and quantitative evaluation metrics to assess the performance of LLMs in the TCM syndrome differentiation thought evaluation task.

This task was presented at the 10th China Health Information Processing Conference, where 239 teams participated in the task, with 17 teams submitting results in the round B. In this paper, we review the evaluation task, the winning teams and their methodologies, and discuss future research directions. Through this work, we aim to contribute valuable insights into LLMs' applicability in TCM and encourage further exploration in this promising intersection of technology and TCM.

2 Related Work

Currently, there is a rapid development of evaluation datasets, such as the MedQA dataset consisting of questions from the US Medical Licensing Examination [11]; the MedM-CQA dataset consisting of questions from the Indian Medical Entrance Examination [12]; the PubMedQA dataset, which includes 1,000 expert-annotated Question-PubMed Abstract-Answer pairs with answers in the form of yes/no/long answer [14]; and the MMLU dataset involving anatomy, clinical medicine, and other disciplines [15]. These benchmarks can be used to evaluate the performance of LLMs from multiple dimensions. With the rapid development of English evaluation datasets, the Chinese evaluation datasets have also been introduced. For example, the Chinese evaluation dataset C-Eval [16] includes a total of 13,948 multiple-choice questions across 52 domains, such as physician qualification, clinical medicine, and basic medicine.

At the same time, several evaluation datasets have been proposed in the field of TCM. For instance, the ShenNong-TCM-EB Evaluation Benchmark (https://github.com/ywj awmw/TCMEB) collects multiple-choice questions related to the Chinese Medicine Practitioner Qualification Examination, covering 16 areas of TCM Basic Theory and TCM Diagnosis. The Qibo-TCM-EB Benchmark includes assessments in three areas: subjective assessment, objective assessment, and TCM NLP tasks [13]. Furthermore, the TCM-ED dataset in TCM-Bench consists of 5,473 questions from the TCM Licensing Examination (TCMLE), including 1,300 questions with authoritative analyses [17]. These specialized datasets are crucial for advancing the evaluation of LLMs in the context of TCM.

3   Dataset

3.1   Overview

Based on the key steps of the TCM syndrome differentiation thought process, an extensive multi-task benchmark was developed to support the application of LLM in TCM. Evaluation task for syndrome differentiation thought of TCM can be divided into the following four subtasks (see Table 1). These subtasks are essential for systematically evaluating different stage of TCM syndrome differentiation.

Table 1. Content of the mandate

Task number	Type of question	Mission statement
Subtask 1	short answer	clinical information extraction
Subtask 2	multiple-choice questions	pathogenesis reasoning
Subtask 3	multiple-choice questions	syndrome reasoning
Subtask 4	short answer	explanatory summary

3.2   Dataset Collection and Annotation

The data in the evolution dataset was annotated by senior TCM students and subsequently reviewed by experienced TCM experts. All annotators and TCM experts were from the Institute of Information on Traditional Chinese Medicine, China Academy of Chinese Medical Sciences and the Institute of Basic Theory for Chinese Medicine, China Academy of Chinese Medical Sciences. Importantly, all annotators had a background in both clinical and informatics aspects of TCM, ensuring the quality and relevance of the annotations.

The task is based on the Baibu knowledge engine [18] tool developed by the project team for manual annotation. We have selected 300 medical case data, including entity annotation, reasoning relationship annotation, and sample data as shown in Table 2.

Table 2. Example data format

Field name	Example
medical record ID	Case 3
clinical Data	Guo, female, 50 years old. Initial diagnosis: June 9, 1983. Chief complaint and medical history: The patient has long suffered from "rheumatic heart disease" and frequently expe-riences palpitations (paroxysmal tachycardia). Due to recurrent episodes, she carries a heavy mental burden, often leading to insomnia. For the past six months, she has often stayed awake all night, sometimes only managing to sleep for 1-2 hours at most, but even then, she is often awakened by nightmares. As a result of long-term insomnia, she experi-ences dizziness, heaviness in the head, mental confusion, and poor appetite. Currently, she is taking western medication, and despite continuously increasing the dosage of various sleeping pills, they have been ineffective. Examination: The patient's complexion is dull, she appears nervous, and has a strong sense of fear. Recently, she has been unable to sleep all night and cannot fall asleep during the day. Her tongue is slightly pale, with a white and greasy coating, and her pulse is thin and weak
clinical information	Dull complexion; nervousness; fear; unable to sleep through the night; slightly pale tongue; thin and weak pulse
answers to TCM pathogenesis	B;C;D
TCM pathogenesis options	A: Fire rising and wind stirring; B: Depletion of qi and blood; C: Insomnia due to gallbladder deficiency; D: Deficiency of heart yin; E: Insufficiency of kidney qi; F: Ob-struction of the mind; G: Internal accumulation of damp-heat; H: Qi deficiency; I: Spleen weakness with dampness predominance; J: Blockage of fetal qi
answers to TCM syndrome	D
TCM syndrome options	A: Damp-heat stagnation; B: Stagnation of blood and heat; C: Stagnation in the chest and epigastric region; D: Deficiency of heart and gallbladder; E: (Repeated) Damp-heat stagna-tion; F: Syndrome of typhoid fever with food retention; G: Accumulation of phlegm and heat; H: Heat scorching the nutritive yin; I: Dampness lingering in the intestines and stom-ach; J: Heat forcing the nutritive blood
explanatory summary	Clinical experience: In this case, due to emotional distress, excessive worry, and strain on the heart and spleen, it led to deficiency of heart yin and depletion of qi and blood, resulting in the spirit being unsettled and insomnia due to gallbladder deficiency. Syndrome differen-tiation: Deficiency of heart and gallbladder

3.3 Dataset Structure

The evaluation dataset contains a total of four sub-tasks of TCM syndrome differentiation and diagnosis problems, including clinical information extraction, TCM pathogenesis reasoning, TCM syndrome reasoning, and explanatory summary. These sub-tasks are crucial for a comprehensive assessment of TCM discursive thinking. The data are divided into training set, validation set, and test set in the ratio of 200:50:50, totaling 300 data. The dataset was provided in JSON format. This structured division allows for effective training and evaluation of the models. The training set, validation set, and test set contain question and label.

4 Submission Result

4.1 Overall Statistics

This evolution dataset serves as the first evaluation task for the CHIP-2024 conference. The evaluation task was released on the Tianchi platform (https://tianchi.aliyun.com/competition/entrance/532222). A total of 239 teams registered this task, among which

47 teams participated in the Round A and 17 teams submitted the results of the Round B. We ranked the teams by calculating the average score of the 17 teams. The top five teams are listed in the Table 3.

Table 3. Top 5 teams and their average score

Team name	Rank	Institution	Avg Score
vvvcx	1	East China Normal University	44.2929
Serendipity	2	Shanghai Jiao Tong University/Xinjiang Medical University	37.5210
Zhijiang IMT	3	Zhijiang Laboratory	35.9954
oi	4	Hohai University	31.9051
Xiansheng	5	Chang'an University	30.9026

4.2 Approach of Top 5

These teams optimized their solutions through various advanced techniques. These included Retrieval Augmented Generation (RAG), instruction tuning, web crawling to build a relevant knowledge base, cue engineering, and fine-tend (QLoRA). Such diverse methods contributed significantly to enhancing the model performance in the evaluation tasks.

The VVVCX team generated 800 pre-trained model tuning data entries rich in localized knowledge and instructions by combining RAG with instruction tuning. This approach significantly enhanced the model's performance in syndrome differentiation thought of TCM. Their innovative methodology highlights the importance of tailored data generation.

The Serendipity team utilized the Baidu_ERNIE_Speed_128K application programming interface (API) and DeepSeekv2 API to generate the final answers. They employed RAG and reordering techniques to optimize the data, significantly enhancing the output accuracy of the model. This demonstrates the effectiveness of integrating multiple tools for improving results.

The Zhijiang IMT team proposed the CotKE-TCM framework, which integrates chain-of-thought and knowledge retrieval enhancement methods, as well as the three necessary medical knowledge resources, to develop an integrated cue engineering system. This comprehensive approach highlights the importance of system integration in TCM applications.

In addition, the Oi team proposed an iterative retrieval-based enhancement generation technique. The Shengsheng team utilized the QLoRA method to fine-tune the Qwen2.5-72B-Instruct model, applying integrated learning techniques to further optimize model performance. These contributions reflect the ongoing innovations in model optimization methodologies.

5   Conclusion

In this paper, we present the TCM syndrome differentiation thought evaluation dataset and provide an overview of the participation in the syndrome differentiation thought evaluation task at the CHIP-2024 conference. This task attracted a large number of participants from both industry and academia, reflecting the growing interest in applying LLMs to TCM.

Following the evaluation, we analyse the methodology used by the winning team, who optimized their approach through an innovative combination of RAG and instruction tuning. Their success highlights the importance of integrating domain-specific knowledge and LLM capabilities to tackle complex reasoning tasks in TCM.

In conclusion, the TCM syndrome differentiation thought evaluation dataset is valuable for enhancing and assessing the reasoning ability of LLMs in the field of TCM. By providing a structured framework for evaluating dialectical reasoning, the dataset offers insights that can guide future improvements in LLMs, particularly in terms in their ability to perform complex reasoning tasks within specialized domains like TCM.

Acknowledgements. This work was supported by Beijing Natural Science Foundation (7252253), Technological Innovation Project of China Academy of Basic Research Operating Expenses Independent Selection Project (ZZ160311), National Natural Science Foundation of China (82174534), Scientific and Technological Innovation Project of China Academy of Chinese Medical Sciences (No. CI2021A05306), National Chinese Medicine Examination 2023 Scientific Research Project (TB2023008).

References

1. Singhal, K., Azizi, S., Tu, T., et al.: Large language models encode clinical knowledge. Nature **620**(7972), 172–180 (2023)
2. Cui, H., Wang, C., Maan, H., et al.: ScGPT: toward building a foundation model for single-cell multi-omics using generative AI. Nat. Methods **21**, 1–11 (2024)
3. Arora, A., Arora, A.: The promise of large language models in health care. Lancet **401**(10377), 641 (2023)
4. Berg, H.T., van Bakel, B., van de Wouw, L., et al.: ChatGPT and generating a differential diagnosis early in an emergency department presentation. Ann. Emerg. Med. **83**(1), 83–86 (2024)
5. McDuff, D., Schaekermann, M., Tu, T., et al.: Towards accurate differential diagnosis with large language models. arXiv preprint arXiv:231200164 (2023)
6. Srivastav, S., Chandrakar, R., Gupta, S., et al.: ChatGPT in radiology: the advantages and limitations of artificial intelligence for medical imaging diagnosis. Cureus **15**(7), e41435 (2023)
7. Liu, H., Azam, M., Bin Naeem, S., et al.: An overview of the capabilities of ChatGPT for medical writing and its implications for academic integrity. Health Inf. Libr. J. **40**(4), 440–446 (2023)
8. Singhal, K., Tu, T., Gottweis, J., et al.: Towards expert-level medical question answering with large language models. arXiv preprint arXiv:230509617 (2023)
9. Peng, C., Yang, X., Chen, A., et al.: A study of generative large language model for medical research and healthcare. NPJ Dig. Med. **6**(1), 210 (2023)

10. Yang, G., Shi, J., Wang, Z., et al.: TCM-GPT: efficient pre-training of large language models for domain adaptation in traditional Chinese medicine. arXiv preprint arXiv:231101786 (2023)
11. Jin, D., Pan, E., Oufattole, N., et al.: What disease does this patient have? A large-scale open domain question answering dataset from medical exams. Appl. Sci. **11**(14), 6421 (2021)
12. Pal, A., Umapathi, L.K., Sankarasubbu, M.: Medmcqa: a large-scale multi-subject multi-choice dataset for medical domain question answering. In: Proceedings of the Conference on Health, Inference, and Learning. PMLR (2022)
13. Zhang, H., Wang, X., Meng, Z., et al.: Qibo: a large language model for traditional Chinese medicine (2024)/ arXiv:2403.16056. https://ui.adsabs.harvard.edu/abs/2024arXiv240 316056Z
14. Jin, Q., Dhingra, B., Liu, Z., et al.: Pubmedqa: a dataset for biomedical research question answering. arXiv preprint arXiv:190906146 (2019)
15. Hendrycks, D., Burns, C., Basart, S., et al.: Measuring massive multitask language understanding. arXiv preprint arXiv:200903300 (2020)
16. Huang, Y., Bai, Y., Zhu, Z., et al.: C-eval: a multi-level multi-discipline chinese evaluation suite for foundation models. Adv. Neural Inf. Process. Syst. **36** (2024)
17. Yue, W., Wang, X., Zhu, W., et al.: TCMBench: a comprehensive benchmark for evaluating large language models in traditional Chinese medicine (2024). arXiv:2406.01126. https://ui. adsabs.harvard.edu/abs/2024arXiv240601126Y
18. Zhang, S., Wang, Z., Yao, K., et al.: The BaiBu knowledge engine: a solution for improving the semantic knowledge base of traditional Chinese medicine. In: Proceedings of the 2023 IEEE International Conference on Bioinformatics and Biomedicine (BIBM), 5–8 December 2023 (2023)

Traditional Chinese Medicine Case Analysis System for High-Level Semantic Abstraction: Optimized with Prompt and RAG

Peng Xu[1], Hongjin Wu[2], Jinle Wang[3(✉)], Rongjia Lin[4], and Liwei Tan[5(✉)]

[1] Chongqing Jiudun Technology Co., Ltd., Chongqing, China
[2] School of Mechanical Science and Engineering, Huazhong University of Science and Technology, Wuhan, China
[3] School of Nursing, Shanghai Jiao Tong University, Shanghai, China
wangjinlee123@163.com
[4] Xinjiang Medical University, Ürümqi, China
[5] School of Mathematical Sciences, Shanghai Jiao Tong University, Shanghai, China
TGS123@sjtu.edu.cn

Abstract. This paper details a technical plan for building a clinical case database for Traditional Chinese Medicine (TCM) using web scraping. Leveraging multiple platforms, including 360doc, we gathered over 5,000 TCM clinical cases, performed data cleaning, and structured the dataset with crucial fields such as patient details, pathogenesis, syndromes, and annotations. Using the *Baidu_ERNIE_Speed_128K* API, we removed redundant information and generated the final answers through the *DeepSeekv2* API, outputting results in standard JSON format. We optimized data recall with Retrieval Augmented Generation(RAG) and rerank techniques during retrieval and developed a hybrid matching scheme. By combining two-stage retrieval method with keyword matching via Jieba, we significantly enhanced the accuracy of model outputs.

Keywords: Rerank · RAG · Jieba

1 Introduction

TCM has been an integral part of Chinese culture for millennia, offering unique diagnostic and therapeutic approaches distinct from Western medicine. Central to TCM is syndrome differentiation, a complex process requiring practitioners to synthesize diverse clinical information to identify underlying pathologies and formulate appropriate treatments. This intricate reasoning process challenges modernization and integration with contemporary medical practices.

Recent developments in Artificial Intelligence (AI), particularly with large language models (LLMs), have shown promising applications in fields requiring complex language understanding and reasoning, including healthcare and

ⓒ The Author(s), under exclusive license to Springer Nature Singapore Pte Ltd. 2025
Y. Zhang et al. (Eds.): CHIP 2024, CCIS 2458, pp. 10–25, 2025.
https://doi.org/10.1007/978-981-96-4298-4_2

TCM. Studies have demonstrated that LLMs such as Zhongjing and Qibo, which are tailored for TCM, can process extensive datasets, uncover underlying patterns, and facilitate new insights into TCM diagnosis and treatment [18]. These AI models can enhance diagnostic accuracy, create standardized treatment approaches, and support integrating traditional practices with modern technological advancements [11, 19].

Several studies have explored the application of AI in TCM. For instance, Yang et al. (2023) introduced Zhongjing, a Chinese medical LLM enhanced through expert feedback and real-world multi-turn dialogues, demonstrating improved capabilities in TCM contexts [18]. Similarly, Zhang et al. (2024) developed Qibo, an LLM tailored for TCM, addressing challenges such as the divergence between TCM theory and modern medicine, and the scarcity of specialized corpora [20]. These efforts underscore the potential of AI to simulate TCM's clinical reasoning processes, thereby elucidating its theoretical framework and facilitating its global dissemination. In addition, community challenges in biomedical text mining have also played a significant role in advancing AI models, providing valuable insights into task evaluation and future research directions [26].

Despite these advancements, challenges remain in developing AI models capable of performing syndrome differentiation with the depth and nuance of experienced TCM practitioners. Existing benchmarks, such as ShenNong-TCM-EB and Qibo-benchmark, primarily focus on basic TCM knowledge and lack the complexity required to evaluate diagnostic reasoning in syndrome differentiation [19]. This gap highlights the need for comprehensive, objective, and systematic evaluation datasets to assess and enhance AI models' capabilities in TCM syndrome differentiation.

Our study aims to construct a high-quality TCM clinical case database tailored to syndrome differentiation reasoning in this context. We collected over 5,000 clinical TCM cases from sources such as 360doc by leveraging web scraping and structured data cleaning techniques. We utilized Baidu's ERNIE Speed 128K API to remove irrelevant information and structure the data into fields, including patient details, syndrome pathology, diagnosis, and treatment notes. For retrieval and reasoning, we implemented hybrid matching schemes combining vector similarity-based matching using gte-Qwen2-1.5B-instruct and keyword matching via jieba segmentation [23], then rerank the results from both retrievers by gte-passage-ranking-multilingual-base [24], achieving improved accuracy and relevance in information retrieval [15, 17]. Answer generation was accomplished using DeepSeekv2 API [5] with prompt optimization, outputting results in JSON format to ensure data standardization.

Our approach also involved testing RAG and rerank techniques, enhancing model responses by integrating initial retrieval results with reordering strategies prioritizing higher-quality outputs. Through these advancements, we constructed a high-quality TCM clinical case database that provides valuable resources for researchers and practitioners while setting a standardized evaluation benchmark for TCM language models.

The remainder of this paper is organized as follows: Sect. 2 reviews related work, highlighting the advancements and challenges in TCM data processing and retrieval. Section 3 outlines the methodology, including data preparation, prompt optimization, and the integration of RAG and Jieba segmentation. Section 4 presents the experimental results, followed by the conclusion in Sect. 5, which summarizes the findings and discusses future directions.

2 Related Work

2.1 Construction of TCM Clinical Case Databases

The construction of clinical case databases in TCM has become increasingly important in facilitating research and practice by standardizing and consolidating clinical information. The China TCM Clinical Case Database by the China Association of Chinese Medicine is one such repository that compiles case studies from renowned TCM experts, aiming to preserve and share TCM knowledge with a broader audience [1,11]. Similarly, studies like those on integrated TCM clinical data platforms focus on managing and analyzing vast amounts of clinical data, providing a structured resource for clinical and research purposes in TCM [11,21].

Our approach builds upon these existing databases by expanding the scope of data sources and integrating advanced retrieval techniques to enhance the accessibility and usability of TCM knowledge [22]. Unlike existing work primarily focusing on case compilation, our system incorporates robust data cleaning, text vectorization, and hybrid retrieval techniques to provide a highly interactive and accurate retrieval experience for TCM practitioners and researchers [19,20].

2.2 Data Cleaning and Structuring for TCM Applications

Data preprocessing, especially data cleaning and structuring, is critical for building high-quality TCM databases. The Chinese Medicine Real-World Data Collection Specification guides data collection methods, database construction, and integration, ensuring high-quality, standardized data across diverse TCM sources [10]. Leveraging such standards, our work utilizes the $Baidu\_ERNIE\_Speed\_128K$ API [14] to harness the understanding capabilities of LLMs. This enables us to perform two critical tasks: first, splitting concatenated low-quality TCM case data into individual cases; and second, filtering out irrelevant information and symbols while extracting essential information, thereby ensuring consistency and quality across the dataset.

Compared to existing efforts focusing on basic data cleaning, our approach also involves structuring TCM case data into essential categories, including patient background, pathogenesis, syndromes, and doctor's notes. This structured format enables a more organized and efficient retrieval process, ensuring TCM researchers can access well-organized data for further analysis and study.

2.3   Hybrid Retrieval Techniques for Enhanced Search Accuracy

Traditional text-based retrieval methods often need to be revised when applied to complex, domain-specific datasets like TCM clinical cases. In response, hybrid retrieval techniques that combine semantic vector similarity with keyword-based matching have gained traction [12]. Studies such as Tencent Cloud's hybrid search applications demonstrate the effectiveness of combining vector-based search with traditional keyword matching to improve search relevance and accuracy [3]. Similarly, Milvus hybrid search tutorials highlight the benefits of integrating dense and sparse vector matching to enhance retrieval precision in specialized fields [2].

Our work builds upon these advancements by utilizing $gte\_Qwen2 - 1.5B - instruct$ [8] for semantic vector generation and Jieba segmentation for keyword extraction, creating a hybrid retrieval system optimised explicitly for TCM data. By combining these methods, our system ensures semantic accuracy and keyword relevance, addressing the unique needs of TCM retrieval. Additionally, we employ RAG techniques [9] and reranking strategies [6] to improve the overall recall and ranking quality, further refining the retrieval process for complex TCM queries.

2.4   TCM Syndrome Differentiation and AI Integration

The core of TCM lies in its diagnostic methodology, particularly syndrome differentiation, which requires practitioners to synthesize a variety of clinical information to identify underlying pathologies and determine the most appropriate treatment strategies. This reasoning process involves not only physiological symptoms but also psychological, emotional, and lifestyle factors, which make TCM diagnosis highly personalized and holistic. Given the complexity and expertise required, this process poses significant challenges for modern AI applications attempting to emulate such nuanced reasoning.

Recent efforts have aimed at bridging this gap by integrating AI into TCM, particularly in automating and simulating syndrome differentiation. Studies such as Hu et al. utilized deep learning models to simulate TCM's diagnostic processes by training models on large clinical datasets. These models demonstrated considerable potential in diagnosing conditions in ways that align with TCM's holistic approach, including considering less quantifiable data such as emotional state or lifestyle factors in diagnosis [7]. Moreover, Zhao et al. developed a knowledge graph-based TCM decision support system, which integrates TCM theory with modern AI technologies. This approach aims to bridge the gap between TCM's theoretical concepts and modern medical practices, providing a framework that could better align TCM with evidence-based medical approaches [25].

2.5   AI Applications in TCM

AI applications in TCM have been rapidly advancing, particularly with the development of systems that assist in diagnosis, treatment recommendation, and personalized healthcare. Recent advancements include the development of LLMs tailored for TCM, which use deep neural networks to understand and process specialized medical knowledge. For example, Zhang et al. introduced Qibo, a Chinese medical LLM, designed to simulate TCM diagnostic reasoning. This model addresses challenges such as the lack of standardized datasets and the complexity of traditional TCM knowledge, making it possible to analyze clinical data more efficiently and accurately [20].

Furthermore, Danielsen et al. implemented a personalized herbal medicine recommendation system using AI, which analyzes patient symptom data to recommend individualized treatments. This is a step forward in using AI not only to understand the symptoms and syndromes but also to propose specific treatments, such as herbal prescriptions, based on patient-specific conditions [4]. Another significant breakthrough in TCM applications is the use of AI-based syndrome differentiation systems, which mimic the diagnostic expertise of TCM practitioners in analyzing complex case data and making treatment decisions. Recent studies like those of Song et al. have shown how combining AI with TCM diagnosis can enhance both the accuracy and efficiency of diagnostic processes [13].

2.6 RAG and Prompt Engineering in NLP

Recent advancements in Natural Language Processing, particularly RAG and Prompt Engineering, have shown significant promise in improving the performance of AI models in complex, specialized fields such as TCM. RAG, which combines information retrieval with generative capabilities, is especially useful in domains where large, dynamic knowledge bases need to be referenced to answer questions or generate text. This hybrid approach has proven to enhance performance in tasks like question answering and text generation, particularly when applied to specialized knowledge areas like medicine and TCM. For example, Lewis et al. demonstrated the success of RAG in the biomedical field, where the integration of information retrieval techniques helped generative models accurately respond to clinical queries by retrieving relevant medical information from external databases [9]. In the context of TCM, RAG has been employed to assist with syndrome differentiation and treatment recommendations, where complex, case-specific knowledge is required to generate accurate and contextually meaningful outputs [25].

In parallel, Prompt Engineering has also made significant strides in recent years. By carefully designing input prompts, researchers can guide large language models to generate more precise and contextually relevant responses, which is crucial for specialized tasks such as medical diagnosis and TCM. Chain-of-Thought (CoT) prompting, as shown in recent work by Wei et al. (2022), has proven to enhance the reasoning accuracy of models in complex domains by encouraging coherent reasoning chains that are essential for tasks requiring detailed, domain-specific knowledge [16]. This technique has been successfully applied to improve the logical accuracy of models in TCM diagnostic tasks. For instance, Yang (2023) developed a prompt engineering framework that allows

AI models to simulate TCM syndrome differentiation by structuring inputs in ways that promote detailed, medically relevant reasoning [18].

Moreover, prompt optimization for medical dialogue systems has demonstrated its utility in refining AI-generated responses, making them more aligned with specific diagnostic frameworks such as those used in TCM. One notable example is the use of the DeepSeekv2 API, which employs optimized prompts to generate high-quality, structured answers in JSON format, adhering to TCM diagnostic standards. This iterative process ensures that generated answers are consistent with TCM practices, providing accurate and reliable responses that can assist TCM practitioners in clinical decision-making [5].

3   Method

3.1   Data Prepare

Data Collection. The data for this study were sourced from multiple reputable TCM knowledge-sharing platforms, including 360doc and other online databases. These platforms provided access to a diverse range of TCM clinical cases, ensuring a comprehensive dataset for analysis. In total, over 5,000 TCM clinical cases were collected to guarantee sufficient breadth and depth of information. The data fields encompass essential attributes such as patient demographics, pathogenesis, syndromes, and commentary, among other critical details, which lay the foundation for subsequent analysis and application.

Data Cleaning and Standardization. To ensure high-quality data, a meticulous data cleaning process was undertaken using the *Baidu_ERNIE _Speed_128K* API. This tool was employed to eliminate redundant and irrelevant information, thereby enhancing the dataset's reliability and usability. Following the cleaning process, the data underwent a comprehensive standardization and structuring phase. This step involved normalizing the field definitions across different data sources to achieve consistency and readability. The result was a well-organized database that meets the requirements of standardized data formats, ensuring compatibility for advanced analyses and machine-learning applications.

Data Integration and Accessibility. The processed and structured database is aligned with academic standards for TCM clinical case studies and serves as a resource for further research and development. The dataset is now hosted and made accessible on a dedicated platform for TCM clinical knowledge, available at TCM Clinical Knowledge Hub. Additionally, to promote open access and reproducibility, the dataset has also been made publicly available via Google Sheets at Open TCM Dataset Repository. This online resource facilitates seamless access for researchers and practitioners interested in exploring diverse TCM clinical case studies, enabling deeper insights into evidence-based TCM practices.

3.2   Chain of Thought

CoT prompting is an effective method to enhance reasoning capabilities in TCM syndrome differentiation by structuring the diagnostic process into clear steps. Starting from clinical information, CoT guides the inference of pathomechanisms and the determination of syndromes through systematic reasoning paths. For instance, given a patient's symptoms such as retrosternal pain, nausea, and acid regurgitation, CoT enables the model to extract key clinical features, infer underlying mechanisms like "stomach disharmony" or "liver qi stagnation" and classify syndromes such as "liver-stomach disharmony" This approach ensures logical and accurate diagnostic outcomes, aligning with the structured thinking required in TCM and improving the model's ability to handle complex causal relationships in diagnosis.

The prompts used in this study are based on DeepSeekv2 API, with structured prompts guiding the model to follow CoT reasoning. A detailed description of the prompt framework is provided in the Appendix 6.

Figure 1 illustrates the difference between a prompt without CoT reasoning and one with CoT in TCM syndrome differentiation tasks. In the "Prompt without CoT" the system repeats the query and fails to infer the implicit relations between clinical information, pathomechanisms, and syndromes, leading to incomplete or incorrect reasoning. In contrast, the "Prompt with CoT" demonstrates step-by-step reasoning, systematically extracting vital clinical features, inferring intermediate pathomechanisms, and deriving the appropriate syndrome classification. This approach enables logical and accurate outputs by explicitly guiding the reasoning process, showcasing how CoT prompting improves interpretability and performance in complex diagnostic tasks.

3.3   Retrieval Augmented Generation

RAG offers a powerful approach to enhancing diagnostic reasoning in TCM by integrating external knowledge retrieval with advanced generative language models. This hybrid methodology addresses the limitations of standalone models by leveraging structured external data to augment the inference process, thereby improving the quality and reliability of diagnostic outputs. The workflow can be shown in Fig. 2.

- **Two-Stage Retrieval Framework.** The RAG framework employs a two-stage retrieval process to extract and rank relevant information from a pre-constructed TCM knowledge base. First, both the user query and the indexed knowledge are vectorized, with similarity-based ranking performed using tools such as FAISS (Facebook AI Similarity Search). The system retrieves a pool of knowledge chunks in the initial stage based on semantic similarity. Subsequently, these initial results are refined through a re-ranking mechanism to prioritize the most contextually relevant information for downstream tasks.
- **Integration with Generative Models.** The retrieved information is incorporated into the generative process by merging it with the user query through

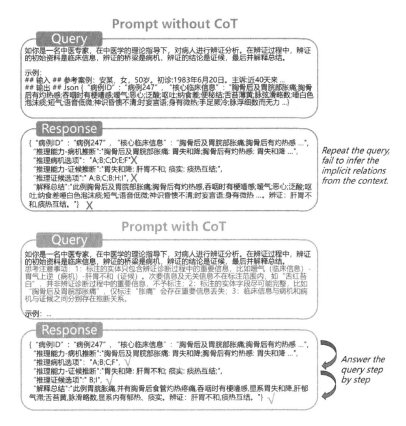

Fig. 1. An example of constructing CoT prompts in the TCM syndrome differentiation task involves integrating reasoning pathways into the diagnostic process. Compared with the original prompt, the CoT prompt adds the corresponding reasoning path for extracting clinical information, inferring pathomechanisms, and determining syndromes before outputting the final diagnosis, ensuring a systematic and logical diagnostic approach.

a structured prompt template. This enriched input is fed into a LLM, enabling it to generate contextually informed responses grounded in domain-specific knowledge.

- **Improved Diagnostic Reasoning.** By incorporating external knowledge, RAG significantly enhances the model's ability to perform complex reasoning tasks, such as pathomechanism inference and syndrome differentiation in TCM. The retrieved information provides a robust foundation for reasoning, ensuring that the outputs—such as the inferred pathomechanism, syndrome classifications, and explanatory summaries-are accurate, interpretable, and aligned with TCM theoretical principles.

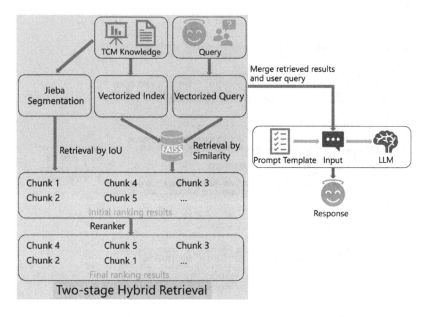

Fig. 2. Illustration of a two-stage retrieval process in a RAG framework for TCM diagnosis, integrating user queries with external knowledge to enhance reasoning and output accuracy.

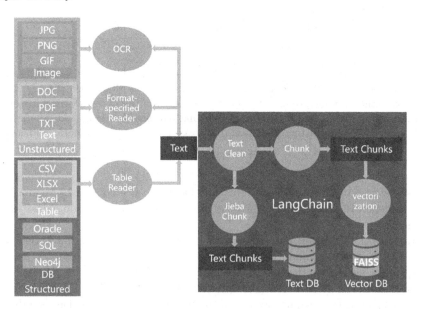

Fig. 3. Comparison of Diagnostic Reasoning with and without RAG in TCM Syndrome Differentiation.

3.4   Jieba Segmentation

In TCM diagnostic tasks, Jieba segmentation is crucial in preprocessing and analyzing textual data, particularly in developing RAG systems. Jieba is a widely used Chinese text segmentation tool that utilizes dictionary-based methods and Hidden Markov Models for accurate word segmentation. It breaks down complex Chinese sentences into meaningful segments, allowing for effective keyword extraction and semantic analysis.

In the workflow illustrated in the Fig. 4 and documentation, Jieba segmentation supports the construction of the TCM knowledge base by enabling precise extraction of key terms such as symptoms, pathomechanisms, and syndromes. By segmenting long and complex clinical texts into manageable entities, Jieba helps enhance the quality of the vectorized query and indexed knowledge. This segmentation, combined with RAG's two-stage retrieval process, improves the relevance and accuracy of retrieved knowledge chunks.

Furthermore, Jieba segmentation enables mixed-matching strategies by integrating IoU-based matching with semantic similarity techniques, as highlighted in the provided materials. This approach ensures that both lexical and contextual nuances of TCM terms are captured, ultimately enhancing the model's ability to perform accurate syndrome differentiation and pathomechanism inference. Through its robust segmentation capabilities, Jieba is a foundational tool in the preprocessing pipeline for TCM-specific RAG systems.

3.5   Demonstration Ranking

The final step in constructing the prompt involves ranking selected demonstrations using a hybrid matching and reranking approach. In our method, we first process both the input query and the cases stored in the database using Jieba segmentation to extract meaningful keywords and semantic units. These are then matched with RAG techniques to identify semantically similar cases from the database. Once an initial ranking is generated, a reranking process is performed to refine the results based on contextual relevance and domain-specific importance. The highest-ranked case from the database, after reranking, is selected and incorporated into the prompt to provide a highly relevant example for the task. This approach ensures that the selected demonstration aligns closely with the input query and enhances the performance of downstream reasoning tasks.

4   Results

4.1   Improving TCM Diagnosis with RAG

The Fig. 3 illustrates the comparative effectiveness of two prompt engineering approaches-one without RAG and the other incorporating RAG-in the context of TCM syndrome differentiation. The results demonstrate that including RAG significantly enhances the model's ability to extract, reason, and infer relationships within the diagnostic process. In the "Prompt without RAG" approach,

Prompt without Rag

Query

如你是一名中医专家，在中医学的理论指导下，对病人进行辨证分析。在辨证过程中，辨证的初始资料是临床信息，辨证的桥梁是病机，辨证的结论是证候，最后并解释总结。

示例：
输入 ## 参考案例：安某，女，50岁。初诊:1983年6月20日。主诉:近40天来 ...
输出 ## Json { "病例ID"："病例247"，"核心临床信息"："胸骨后及胃脘部胀痛;胸骨后有灼热感;吞咽时有梗噎感;嗳气;恶心;泛酸;呕吐;纳食差;便秘结;舌苔薄黄;脉弦滑略数;唾白色泡沫痰;短气;语音低微;神识昏愦不清;时妄言语;身有微热;手足厥冷;脉浮细数而无力 ...}

Response

{ "病例ID"："病例247"，"核心临床信息"："胸骨后及胃脘部胀痛;胸骨后有灼热感 ...",
    "推理能力-病机推断":"胸骨后及胃脘部胀痛: 胃失和降;胸骨后有灼热感: 胃失和降 ...",
    "推理病机选项"："A;B;C;D;E;F" ✗
    "推理能力-证候推断":"胃失和降: 肝胃不和; 痰实: 痰热互结;",
    "推理证候选项":" A;B;C;H;I", ✗
    "解释总结":"此例胸骨后及胃脘部胀痛;胸骨后有灼热感,吞咽时有梗噎感;嗳气;恶心;泛酸;呕吐;纳食差唾白色泡沫痰;短气;语音低微;神识昏愦不清;时妄言语;身有微热 ...。辨证: 肝胃不和,痰热互结。"} ✗

Repeat the query, fail to infer the implicit relations from the context.

Prompt with Rag

Query

如你是一名中医专家，在中医学的理论指导下，对病人进行辨证分析。在辨证过程中，辨证的初始资料是临床信息，辨证的桥梁是病机，辨证的结论是证候，最后并解释总结。

示例：
输入 ## 参考案例：安某，女，50岁。初诊:1983年6月20日。主诉:近40天来...+诊查:现面色无华，舌质淡红，舌苔薄黄，脉弦滑略数，经钡餐透视检查诊为可复性食管裂孔疝，反流性食管炎。辨证:肝胃不和，痰热互结(RAG)。
输出 ## Json { "病例ID"："病例247"，"核心临床信息"："胸骨后及胃脘部胀痛;胸骨后有灼热感;吞咽时有梗噎感;嗳气;恶心;泛酸;呕吐;纳食差;便秘结;舌苔薄黄;脉弦滑略数;唾白色泡沫痰;短气;语音低微;神识昏愦不清;时妄言语;身有微热;手足厥冷;脉浮细数而无力 ...}

Response

{ "病例ID"："病例247"，"核心临床信息"："胸骨后及胃脘部胀痛;胸骨后有灼热感 ...",
    "推理能力-病机推断":"胸骨后及胃脘部胀痛: 胃失和降;胸骨后有灼热感: 胃失和降 ...",
    "推理病机选项"："A;B;C;F", √
    "推理能力-证候推断":"胃失和降: 肝胃不和; 痰实: 痰热互结;",
    "推理证候选项":" B;I", √
    "解释总结":"此例胃脘胀痛,并有胸骨后食管灼热绞痛,吞咽时有梗噎感,显系胃失和降,肝郁气滞;舌苔黄,脉滑略数,显系内有郁热、痰实。辨证: 肝胃不和,痰热互结。"} √

Answer the query step by step

Fig. 4. Illustration of a preprocessing pipeline for structured and unstructured data, integrating OCR, text cleaning, jieba chunking, text segmentation, and vectorization for creating a searchable hybrid database.

the model struggles to infer implicit relationships from the context and often repeats the input query without generating meaningful or logically coherent responses. For instance, in the example provided, the model incorrectly selects options for "pathogenesis reasoning" and provides a summary that lacks depth and alignment with TCM principles. This demonstrates the limitations of relying solely on the model's internal knowledge, as it fails to address the complexity of the task. Conversely, the "Prompt with RAG" approach leverages external knowledge retrieval to supplement the model's reasoning process. By integrating relevant TCM case data and knowledge, the model can systematically extract clinical information, perform accurate pathogenesis and syndrome differentiation, and provide a well-structured, step-by-step explanation. For example, the model correctly identifies the relationships between clinical symptoms, Pathogenesis ("stomach disharmony and impaired descending" and "liver qi stagnation") and syndromes ("liver-stomach disharmony" and "phlegm-heat accumulation"), demonstrating improved reasoning accuracy and alignment with TCM diagnostic principles.

4.2   Effect of RAG and Jieba Segmentation

The results in Table 1 demonstrate the comparative performance between naive overlap window and hybrid method with Jieba in handling TCM dataset tasks. While both methods show competitive results, Jieba slightly outperforms overlap window with a score of 37.05 compared to 36.15. Jieba Segmentation: The higher score achieved by Jieba suggests its advantage in keyword-based matching tasks. Jieba's ability to perform efficient tokenization of Chinese text likely contributes to its strong performance in this context. RAG: Although slightly behind Jieba, RAG performed well with a score of 36.15, showcasing its effectiveness in leveraging semantic retrieval. RAG's ability to retrieve contextually relevant information might make it more suitable for tasks requiring deeper semantic understanding. The comparison highlights that while Jieba excels in tasks dependent on accurate tokenization and keyword matching, RAG's strength lies in semantic-driven retrieval. This suggests potential benefits in combining both methods to achieve optimal results, leveraging Jieba's precision in segmentation and RAG's contextual retrieval capabilities.

Table 1. Comparison of Scores for Different Text Segmentation Methods

Method	Score
Naive RAG	36.15
Naive RAG + Jieba	37.05

4.3   Performance Comparison of LLMs in TCM Clinical Reasoning

Based on the document provided, the experimental section emphasizes leveraging various AI models to process and analyze Chinese medicine clinical case data.

Table 2. Comparison of Scores for Different Models (Base Version Test)

Model	Access	Score
GPT-4o	API	25.62
DeepSeekV2	API	27.38
Qwen2-72B	Local	25.32
GLM-4	API	24.13
Baidu-ERNIE-Speed-128K	API	26.16

The comparison of different base models highlights their respective performance across tasks, particularly focusing on classification and data generation accuracy.

The experiments shown in Table 2 evaluated the performance of several base models on specific tasks involving TCM clinical reasoning and dataset analysis. The models were tested using structured and cleaned TCM data from various sources, including over 5,000 case records. Advanced AI techniques, such as prompt optimization and mixed retrieval methods, were employed to enhance performance. Among the tested models: DeepSeekV2 achieved the highest score of 27.38, reflecting its strong ability to handle structured TCM data and classification tasks effectively. ERNIE (26.16) and GPT-4o (25.62) also demonstrated competitive results, albeit slightly less effective than DeepSeekV2. Qwen2-72B scored 25.32, showing moderate efficiency in semantic understanding and classification. GLM-4, with a score of 24.13, lagged slightly behind the other models, indicating room for improvement in handling TCM-specific data.

The experimental results suggest that DeepSeekV2 is better suited for tasks requiring nuanced interpretation of TCM data, potentially due to its prompt engineering and fine-tuned parameters. Future work will focus on refining model inputs, enhancing retrieval accuracy, and expanding the dataset to improve generalizability and performance across models.

5   Conclusion

This study presents a comprehensive framework for enhancing TCM syndrome differentiation through advanced AI techniques, focusing on integrating RAG and Jieba segmentation. By leveraging over 5,000 structured clinical cases and optimizing prompts with the DeepSeekV2 API, the research has demonstrated significant improvements in the accuracy and relevance of diagnostic reasoning. Key findings highlight that including RAG enables models to retrieve and utilize external domain-specific knowledge, thereby overcoming the limitations of standalone generative models. Combining vector-based semantic matching (gte_Qwen2-1.5B-instruct), keyword extraction (Jieba segmentation) and reranker (gte-passage-ranking-multilingual-base), the two-stage hybrid retrieval approach ensures precise and contextually rich outputs. Moreover, the step-by-step reasoning enabled by CoT prompts further aligns diagnostic outputs with TCM principles, enhancing interpretability and reliability. Comparative experiments reveal that RAG significantly enhances reasoning tasks, improving the inference of pathogenesis and syndrome classification accuracy. For instance, the RAG-based approach successfully identifies critical relationships, such as linking "stomach disharmony" and "liver qi stagnation" with "liver-stomach disharmony" and "phlegm-heat accumulation." Additionally, performance comparisons between segmentation methods indicate that Jieba excels in token-based tasks, while RAG provides a deeper semantic understanding, suggesting the complementary nature of these techniques. This research establishes a robust methodological foundation for modernizing TCM diagnosis through AI. Developing a standardized TCM case database and retrieval-enhanced reasoning models contributes to bridging traditional diagnostic practices with contemporary computational methodologies. Future work should explore expanding the dataset, integrating multi-modal data (e.g., imaging and lab reports), and refining retrieval mechanisms further to enhance the generalizability and efficacy of AI-assisted TCM diagnostics. This progress benefits the scientific understanding of TCM and fosters its global dissemination and integration into modern healthcare systems.

6   Appendix: Prompt for TCM Syndrome Differentiation

The following prompt is used for TCM syndrome differentiation, where the model simulates the process of diagnosis based on clinical information and performs reasoning to infer the disease mechanisms and the syndrome. The prompt guides the model through the steps of extracting key clinical features, reasoning the pathomechanisms, and determining the syndrome.

task_all = """如你是一名中医专家，在中医学的理论指导下，对病人进行辨证分析。在辨证过程中，辨证的初始资料是临床信息，辨证的桥梁是病机，辨证的结论是证候，解释总结是对整个辨证过程的总结。
请参考案例的识别、抽取、推断方法对实际案例进行诊断分析，要求输出必须包括：
    * 病例ID
    * 核心临床信息
    * 推理能力-病机推断
    * 推理病机选项
    * 推理能力-证候推断
    * 推理证候选项
    * 解释总结:
概念说明：
    临床信息：中医师在进行辨证诊断过程中，从患者的临床资料中提取出临床信息，包括患者的症状、体征、病史等
    病机：在辨证诊断过程中，中医师根据患者的临床信息，通过逐步推理的关于疾病本质和关键病理变化的结论。
    证候：在病机的基础上，进一步推断出的患者当前病情的主要证候类型。
思考注意事项：
    1：标注的实体只包含辨证诊断过程中的重要信息，比如嗳气（临床信息）-胃气上逆（病机）-肝胃不和（证候）。次要信息及无关信息不在标注范围内，如\舌红苔白"，并非辨证诊断过程中的重要信息，不予标注。
    2：标注的实体字段尽可能完整，比如\胸骨后及胃脘部胀痛"，仅标注\胀痛"会存在重要信息丢失。
    3：临床信息与病机和病机与证候之间分别存在推断关系

特别重要：
    为帮助理解，我会输入参考案例，你要将其作为参考资料，从中可以提取你需要的信息，包括核心临床信息，病机，推理和解释总结。

具体步骤:

从参考案例中提取精确匹配到的案例，如果提取到，具体为，日期，主诉及病史保持一致。则为精确匹配，参考案例中的病机，证候 将直接用于选项的匹配。如果没有精确匹配，则根据参考案例，依靠自己的能力对输入的实际案例按照顺序 核心临床信息提取-->推理能力-病机推断-->推理病机选项-->推理能力-证候推断-->推理证候选项-->解释总结 进行诊断分析。
""""

This prompt is used in the task of simulating the syndrome differentiation process in TCM. The output requires detailed information about the clinical case, disease mechanisms, syndrome, and an overall diagnostic explanation. The instructions guide the model to extract relevant clinical information, perform reasoning, and generate the necessary diagnostic steps.

References

1. Line spacing in latex documents. https://www.popsci.com/article/technology/how-will-drones-change-sports/
2. Batifol, S.: Getting started with hybrid search with milvus. https://zilliz.com/blog/hybrid-search-with-milvus
3. Csakash: Hybrid search a method to optimize rag implementation. https://medium.com/@csakash03/hybrid-search-is-a-method-to-optimize-rag-implementation-98d9d0911341
4. Danielsen, S., Davidson, E., Fredrickson, G., Segalman, R.: Absence of electrostatic rigidity in conjugated polyelectrolytes with pendant charges. ACS Macro Lett. 8(9), 1147–1152 (2019). https://doi.org/10.1021/acsmacrolett.9b00551
5. DeepSeek-AI, et al.: DeepSeek-V2: a strong, economical, and efficient mixture-of-experts language model. arXiv e-prints arXiv:2405.04434 (2024). https://doi.org/10.48550/arXiv.2405.04434
6. Gao, J., et al.: LLM-enhanced reranking in recommender systems. arXiv e-prints arXiv:2406.12433 (2024). https://doi.org/10.48550/arXiv.2406.12433
7. Hu, H., Li, Y., Zheng, Z., Hu, W., Lin, R., Kang, Y.: A traditional Chinese medicine prescription recommendation model based on contrastive pre-training and hierarchical structure network. Expert Syst. Appl. 126318 (2025). https://doi.org/10.1016/j.eswa.2024.126318. https://www.sciencedirect.com/science/article/pii/S0957417424031853
8. Hui, B., et al.: Qwen2.5-coder technical report. arXiv e-prints arXiv:2409.12186 (2024). https://doi.org/10.48550/arXiv.2409.12186
9. Lewis, P., et al.: Retrieval-augmented generation for knowledge-intensive NLP tasks. arXiv e-prints arXiv:2005.11401 (2020). https://doi.org/10.48550/arXiv.2005.11401
10. Li, X., et al.: Ltm-tcm: a comprehensive database for the linking of traditional Chinese medicine with modern medicine at molecular and phenotypic levels. Pharmacol. Res. **178**, 106185 (2022). https://doi.org/10.1016/j.phrs.2022.106185
11. Ren, M., Huang, H., Zhou, Y., Cao, Q., Bu, Y., Gao, Y.: TCM-SD: a benchmark for probing syndrome differentiation via natural language processing. arXiv e-prints arXiv:2203.10839 (2022). https://doi.org/10.48550/arXiv.2203.10839

12. Sarmah, B., Hall, B., Rao, R., Patel, S., Pasquali, S., Mehta, D.: HybridRAG: integrating knowledge graphs and vector retrieval augmented generation for efficient information extraction. arXiv e-prints arXiv:2408.04948 (2024). https://doi.org/10.48550/arXiv.2408.04948
13. Song, Y., Ma, S., Dai, Y., Lu, J.: Ai-assisted tcm syndrome differentiation: key issues and technical challenges. Strat. Study CAE **26**, 234 (2024). https://doi.org/10.15302/J-SSCAE-2024.02.010
14. Sun, Y., et al.: ERNIE: enhanced representation through knowledge integration. arXiv e-prints arXiv:1904.09223 (2019). https://doi.org/10.48550/arXiv.1904.09223
15. Webb, N.A., et al.: Gender and precarity in astronomy. In: Journées 2022 de la Société Française d'Astronomie & d'Astrophysique (2023)
16. Wei, J., et al.: Chain-of-thought prompting elicits reasoning in large language models. arXiv e-prints arXiv:2201.11903 (2022). https://doi.org/10.48550/arXiv.2201.11903
17. Weisz, J.D., Muller, M., He, J., Houde, S.: Toward general design principles for generative AI applications. arXiv e-prints arXiv:2301.05578 (2023). https://doi.org/10.48550/arXiv.2301.05578
18. Yang, S., et al.: Zhongjing: enhancing the Chinese medical capabilities of large language model through expert feedback and real-world multi-turn dialogue. arXiv e-prints arXiv:2308.03549 (2023). https://doi.org/10.48550/arXiv.2308.03549
19. Yue, W., et al.: TCMBench: a comprehensive benchmark for evaluating large language models in traditional Chinese medicine. arXiv e-prints arXiv:2406.01126 (2024). https://doi.org/10.48550/arXiv.2406.01126
20. Zhang, H., et al.: Qibo: a large language model for traditional Chinese medicine. arXiv e-prints arXiv:2403.16056 (2024). https://doi.org/10.48550/arXiv.2403.16056
21. Zhang, P., Shen, S., Deng, W., Mao, S., Wang, Y.: The construction model of the tcm clinical knowledge coding database based on knowledge organization. BioMed Res. Int. **2022**, 1–7 (2022). https://doi.org/10.1155/2022/2503779
22. Zhang, T., Huang, Z., Wang, Y., Wen, C., Peng, Y., Ye, Y.: Information extraction from the text data on traditional Chinese medicine: a review on tasks, challenges, and methods from 2010 to 2021. Evidence-based complementary and alternative medicine: eCAM **2022**, 1679589 (2022)
23. Zhang, X., Wu, P., Cai, J., Wang, K.: A contrastive study of Chinese text segmentation tools in marketing notification texts. J. Phys. Conf. Ser. **1302**, 022010 (2019). https://doi.org/10.1088/1742-6596/1302/2/022010
24. Zhang, X., et al.: mgte: generalized long-context text representation and reranking models for multilingual text retrieval. arXiv preprint arXiv:2407.19669 (2024)
25. Zhao, X., et al.: The construction of a tcm knowledge graph and application of potential knowledge discovery in diabetic kidney disease by integrating diagnosis and treatment guidelines and real-world clinical data. Front. Pharmacol. **14**, 1147677 (2023)
26. Zong, H., et al.: Advancing Chinese biomedical text mining with community challenges. J. Biomed. Inf. **157**, 104716 (2024). https://doi.org/10.1016/j.jbi.2024.104716

A TCM Syndrome Differentiation Thinking Method Based on Chain of Thought and Knowledge Retrieval Augmentation

Jianfeng Zhang[1], Xiang Li[3], Jian Fang[1], Wenqi Wei[1], and Menglin Cui[2(✉)]

[1] Zhejiang Lab, Hangzhou, China
{zhangjianfeng,jianfang,weiwq}@zhejianglab.org
[2] Business School, University of Shanghai for Science and Technology, Shanghai, China
mcui@usst.edu.cn
[3] AI Innovation Department, ANTA Group, Xiamen, China

Abstract. With the advent of large language models (LLMs), evaluating their diagnostic thinking abilities is gaining much consideration in the field of traditional Chinese medicine (TCM). Within this context, we propose an innovative framework named CotKE-TCM, which integrates chain-of-thought and knowledge retrieval enhancement methodologies for TCM diagnostic thinking. This framework integrates three essential medical knowledge resources: 1) acquiring case knowledge through case similarity analysis to offer intuitive reference cases for TCM diagnosis; 2) leveraging LLMs to produce specialized TCM knowledge, guiding the model towards a more accurate understanding of disease causality and syndrome differentiation; 3) obtaining clinical experience knowledge via retrieval techniques to effectively complement the limitations inherent in training data. By skillfully combining these three knowledge sources, we have developed a comprehensive prompting engineering system. The experimental outcomes demonstrate exceptional performance on the final test dataset provided by the 10th China Health Informatics Processing Conference (CHIP 2024). This not only verifies the efficacy of the CotKE-TCM framework but also provides significant references and insights for the future advancement of intelligent TCM.

Keywords: Large Language Models · Traditional Chinese Medicine · TCM Diagnosis · Retrieval Enhancement · Chain-of-Thought

1 Introduction

Traditional Chinese Medicine (TCM), refined over thousands of years of empirical testing and practical experience, stands as a vital component of contemporary medical science and plays a pivotal role in promoting human health [1,2]. Nevertheless, elucidating the scientific foundations of TCM in a way that is both

© The Author(s), under exclusive license to Springer Nature Singapore Pte Ltd. 2025
Y. Zhang et al. (Eds.): CHIP 2024, CCIS 2458, pp. 26–38, 2025.
https://doi.org/10.1007/978-981-96-4298-4_3

accessible and engaging poses a significant challenge in the ongoing effort to modernize this ancient practice.

With the rapid advancement of artificial general intelligence, large language models (LLMs) have demonstrated impressive abilities in natural language understanding [3,4], generation [5,6] and reasoning [7–9]. These pre-trained models can process and comprehend vast amounts of data, learning and discovering potential knowledge, thus providing a powerful platform for research and application in TCM. Despite their numerous achievements across various domains, even the most cutting-edge LLMs are susceptible to generating information that is either inaccurate or illogical-a phenomenon referred to as 'hallucinations' [10,11]. Such inaccuracies present considerable risks when integrating LLMs into real-world scenarios. To mitigate these challenges, Retrieval-Augmented Generation (RAG) [12] has emerged as a promising solution, enhancing the factual accuracy of generated content by incorporating pertinent information from external knowledge bases into the model's output process [13–15]. Motivated by this approach, we introduce CotKE-TCM, an innovative TCM dialectical thinking framework that integrates chain-of-thought reasoning with knowledge retrieval enhancements.

The main contributions of this paper are summarized as follows:

1. We designed a knowledge integration framework that merges three types of key medical knowledge resources: case knowledge obtained through case similarity analysis, TCM professional knowledge generated using LLMs, and clinical experience knowledge acquired through retrieval technology.
2. We adopted a TCM dialectical thinking chain approach to guide the large model to reason according to the principles of TCM dialectical thinking.
3. Our proposed method achieved commendable results in the TCM dialectical thinking evaluation.

2   Related Works

2.1   Large Language Models

LLMs refer to language models based on transformer architecture with hundreds of billions (or more) parameters, trained on large-scale text data, such as GPT-3 [16], PaLM [17], Alactica [18], and LLaMA [19]. LLMs have demonstrated strong capabilities in understanding natural language and solving complex tasks through text generation. Due to their pre-training on mixed-source corpora, they can capture rich knowledge from large-scale pre-training data, potentially becoming experts in specific domains. Additionally, through instruction fine-tuning and alignment fine-tuning, they can conveniently adapt to areas where their performance is suboptimal. Research shows that LLMs can promote the development of multiple fields, including healthcare, education, finance, and scientific research [20].

Despite their remarkable performance, LLMs can be further improved through a simple strategy called In-Context Learning (ICL) [21]. ICL aims to enhance model performance by editing prompts. It uses formatted natural language prompts containing task descriptions and/or several task examples as demonstrations. The reason ICL works is that LLMs possess the ability to learn from a few examples, meaning they can achieve good results on new tasks without additional training or gradient updates by providing a few demonstrations [21].

2.2   Chain-of-Thought

Chain-of-Thought (CoT) [22] is an emerging artificial intelligence method aimed at enhancing the capabilities of machine learning models by simulating the human thought process when solving complex problems. The core of the CoT method lies in breaking down the problem-solving process into a series of logical steps or thought links, each of which includes further analysis and reasoning based on the output from the previous step, gradually approaching the final answer. This method not only improves the accuracy of the model in solving problems but also enhances the transparency and explainability of its decision-making process, which is particularly important for applications requiring high trust, such as healthcare.

In TCM dialectical thinking, the application of CoT is especially crucial [23, 24]. TCM diagnosis emphasizes the combination of "observation, auscultation and olfaction, inquiry, and palpation," requiring doctors to make comprehensive judgments based on the patient's specific symptoms and signs, combined with personal experience and theoretical knowledge. This process is essentially a complex, multi-step reasoning process, making it highly suitable for modeling using the CoT method. By explicitly representing each step of the dialectical process, CoT can help AI systems better understand and learn the diagnostic logic of TCM experts, while also promoting non-experts understanding of TCM theory and increasing acceptance of treatment plans.

2.3   Retrieval-Augmented Generation

RAG [12] is a model that combines retrieval and generation techniques. It generates answers or content by referencing information from external knowledge bases, offering strong interpretability and customization capabilities. RAG serves as a complementary approach to overcome knowledge limitations. It adopts a retrieve-then-read process, integrating relevant documents from external knowledge sources into the generation process of LLMs [13–15]. Suitable for various natural language processing tasks, including question-answering systems, document generation, and intelligent assistants, RAG models excel in their versatility, enabling real-time knowledge updates and providing more efficient and precise information services through end-to-end evaluation methods [25].

3   Methodology

To achieve the TCM dialectical thinking task, we propose an innovative TCM dialectical thinking framework named CotKE-TCM, which combines chain-of-thought with knowledge retrieval enhancement. In Sect. 3.1, we introduce the basic situation of the TCM dialectical thinking task. In Sect. 3.2, we construct a TCM dialectical thinking chain, including reasoning paths from clinical information to disease mechanisms and from disease mechanisms to syndromes. In Sect. 3.3, we introduce the knowledge retrieval enhancement framework, which integrates three types of critical medical knowledge resources: case knowledge obtained through case similarity analysis, TCM professional knowledge generated using LLMs, and clinical experience knowledge acquired through retrieval technology. In Sect. 3.4, we organically combine these intermediate results to generate a prompt, call the large model, and perform final data format processing (see Fig. 1).

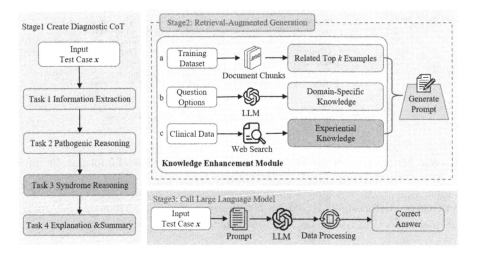

Fig. 1. Overall Research Framework. Stage 1 constructs the reasoning process from clinical information to disease mechanisms and from disease mechanisms to syndromes. Stage 2 utilizes knowledge retrieval enhancement technology to integrate three types of TCM knowledge. Stage 3 organically combines the knowledge to construct a prompt template, call the large model, and perform data processing.

3.1 Task Introduction

The TCM dialectical thinking process involves a comprehensive analysis of various clinical data under the guidance of TCM theory, leading to the extraction of disease mechanisms and the summarization into complete syndrome names. Based on the TCM dialectical thinking process, we identify four key steps, as shown in Fig. 2.

Clinical Information Recognition and Extraction: Based on the textual information of the case, recognize and extract clinical information, including general symptoms, tongue and pulse conditions, causes, and examination results.

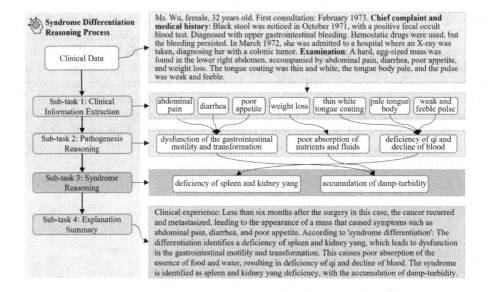

Fig. 2. Key Steps of the Dialectical Thinking Process.

Disease Mechanism Inference: Using the extracted clinical information, infer the disease mechanism.

Syndrome Inference: Based on the inferred disease mechanism, determine the final dialectical result, i.e., the syndrome.

Explanation and Summary: Integrate the above steps to explain and summarize the dialectical thinking process, including clinical insights and the dialectical result.

According to the requirements of the organizers, the reasoning process is divided into four sub-tasks. For given clinical information and related materials, the logical reasoning work for sub-tasks 1 to 4 must be completed in sequence, and the order cannot be adjusted, as shown in Table 1.

3.2   Constructing the TCM Dialectical Thinking Chain

CoT prompts have been proven to effectively enhance the reasoning capabilities of LLMs in both zero-shot settings and few-shot ICL settings [22]. Next, we provide a detailed explanation of how to derive the specific reasoning paths in the TCM dialectical thinking task.

As shown in Fig. 3, the TCM dialectical thinking process is illustrated using an example of inferring disease mechanisms from clinical information. In the original input, the model input includes a description of the task type, with examples 1 to n selected from the training data as valuable demonstrations. Example $n+1$ is a real query from a TCM test case, and the model output is the

Table 1. Content of the Syndrome Differentiation Task.

Task	Question Type	Example Questions
Sub-task 1	Short Answer	Identify and extract clinical information from the question, following the"Clinical Information" format in the example.
Sub-task 2	Multiple Choice	Following the "Pathogenesis Reasoning (Clinical Information → Pathogenesis)" format in the example, select the correct pathogenesis(s) from the options (multiple answers allowed): A: Spleen-Kidney Yang Deficiency; B: Yangming Heat; C: Lower Deficiency-Upper Excess; D: Latent Wind in Lung; E: Qi-Blood Depletion; F: Qi-Fluid Damage from Excessive Sweating; G: Dysfunction of Gastrointestinal Transport; H: Phlegm-Heat Transformation; I: Poor Absorption of Nutrients; J: Liver Qi Transverse Invasion
Sub-task 3	Multiple Choice	Following the "Pathogenesis Reasoning (Clinical Information → Pathogenesis)" format in the example, select the correct pathogenesis(s) from the options (multiple answers allowed): A: Damp-Heat; B: Internal Phlegm-Fire; C: Liver-Kidney Deficiency; D: Phlegm-Heat Disturbing Spirit; E: Internal Liver Wind; F: Obstruction of Nutrient-Defense; G: Spleen Failing to Control Blood; H: Spleen-Kidney Yang Deficiency; I: Internal Liver Wind; J: Damp-Turbidity Accumulation
Sub-task 4	Short Answer	Write clinical insights and diagnostic conclusions summarizing the diagnostic process, following the "Interpretation & Summary" format in the example.

selection of a disease mechanism from the provided options. However, the model does not fully understand the underlying semantic relationships between clinical data, clinical information, and disease mechanism results, leading to biased outcomes. To address this issue, we provide the model with specific reasoning paths from clinical information to disease mechanisms and from disease mechanisms to syndromes (Fig. 1, Stage 1). This approach ultimately achieves correct results and enhances the model's performance.

3.3 TCM-Informed Retrieval Enhancement

The Retrieval-Augmented Generation (RAG) model combines language models with information retrieval techniques. When the model needs to generate text or answer questions, it first retrieves relevant information from a large document collection and then uses this retrieved information to guide text generation, thereby improving the quality and accuracy of predictions.

Randomly selecting training data as examples can improve model performance, but this method is unstable and may lead to performance degradation. Additionally, the training set provided by the organizers cannot cover all clinical cases in the test set. Therefore, we propose a TCM dialectical thinking framework that integrates similarity retrieval and domain knowledge enhancement, as shown in Fig. 1, Stage 2.

3.3.1 Similarity-Based Demonstration Selection Selecting appropriate demonstrations from the training set to guide the LLM in performing high-quality reasoning for test texts is crucial. In this step, we adopt a method of retrieving documents related to the test data, which significantly enhances model

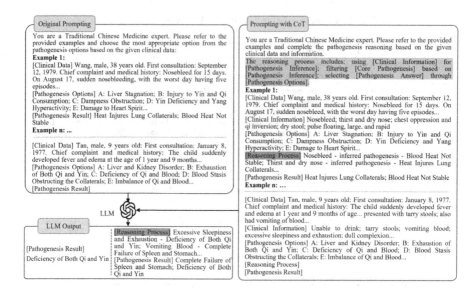

Fig. 3. An example of constructing a Cot prompt in the TCM dialectical thinking-disease mechanism inference task. Compared to the original prompt, the Cot prompt adds the corresponding reasoning path before outputting the label for each demonstration.

performance. We use the Graph-based Text Embedding (BGE) method [26]. BGE maps text data into a low-dimensional space for retrieval and similarity calculation. It focuses on the semantic structure of text data and provides better semantic relevance. In this paper, we use the bge-base-zh-v1.5 model to compute the output vectors of all data in the training set for retrieval.

As shown in Fig. 1, Stage 2a, we calculate the cosine similarity between the representation vector of the current input sentence and the retrieval vectors of the training set data, and select the top n data with the highest similarity as demonstrations. Then, we rank the training data in descending order of similarity scores as demonstrations 1-n. Both the test samples and training samples are pure clinical data texts with basic information removed.

3.3.2 LLM-Based Option Knowledge Enhancement

Tasks 2 and 3 (disease mechanism and syndrome inference) are the most critical modules in the TCM dialectical thinking evaluation. These modules require the model to select one or more correct options from the given case options as answers. Each option often contains rich medical knowledge and clinical experience, which are crucial for the test taker's understanding and judgment. To improve the accuracy and depth of understanding in answering, we propose an LLM-based option knowledge enhancement method, as shown in Fig. 1, Stage 2b.

We use LLMs to parse the content of each option and supplement relevant TCM knowledge points. This includes overviews, etiology and pathogenesis, clinical manifestations, and diagnostic key points. The purpose of this step is to provide more comprehensive background information, helping the test taker build a complete knowledge framework. For example, for the option "Liver Qi Stagnation", the LLM can supplement the following knowledge points:

Liver Qi Stagnation: A TCM term referring to a dysfunction of the liver leading to impaired qi circulation. Common symptoms include emotional depression, chest and rib pain, belching, etc. It often occurs in situations of emotional distress and excessive stress.

Etiology and Pathogenesis: The liver is responsible for free flow. Emotional distress and excessive stress can lead to liver qi stagnation, which in turn affects qi circulation, resulting in qi stagnation.

Clinical Manifestations: Emotional depression, chest and rib pain, belching, loss of appetite, menstrual irregularities, etc.

Diagnostic Key Points: Diagnosis is made through a comprehensive judgment based on medical history, observation of the tongue and pulse, and the patient's clinical manifestations.

3.3.3 Retrieval-Based Experiential Knowledge Enhancement In addition to enhancing options with knowledge using LLMs, we can further enrich the model's prompt information by further calling web searches to retrieve similar historical cases, as shown in Fig. 1, Stage 2c. This method not only provides more clinical experience and real-world cases but also helps the model better understand the background and complexity of the questions. The implementation steps for retrieval-based experiential knowledge enhancement are as follows:

Keyword Extraction: Extract key symptoms, signs, and diagnostic information from the given case to form search keywords.

Similar Case Retrieval: Use search engines (such as Baidu, Google, etc.) to input the extracted keywords and retrieve related clinical cases and literature. Screening and Organization: Screen the search results to identify historical cases similar to the given case and extract key information.

Experiential Knowledge Summary: Summarize the extracted key information to form experiential knowledge. This experiential knowledge can include common diagnostic approaches, effective treatment methods, potential complications, and their management strategies.

By incorporating this experiential knowledge, the model can gain a deeper understanding of the clinical context and make more accurate and informed decisions.

3.4 Data Integration and Processing

In the previous stages, we have generated multiple intermediate results using various methods, such as similarity-based demonstration selection, LLM-based option knowledge enhancement, and retrieval-based experiential knowledge enhancement. To generate the final prompt template, these intermediate results need to be organically combined to form a complete and coherent input, as shown in Fig. 4. The entire process is described as follows:

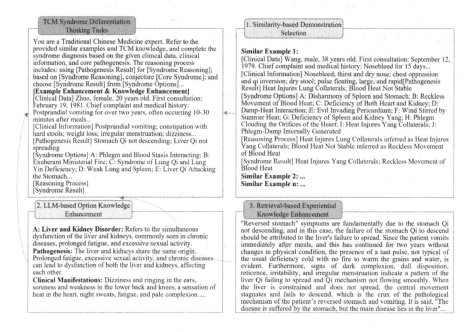

Fig. 4. Organically combine the intermediate results generated by various methods to create the final prompt template.

Adding Reasoning Paths: According to the CoT method, add detailed reasoning paths for each step to the prompt to help the model better understand the task requirements.

Retrieval-Augmented Knowledge: Embed the disease mechanism and syndrome knowledge points generated by LLMs and the experiential knowledge obtained through retrieval into the prompt, providing rich background information and clinical experience.

Constructing the Final Prompt: Combine all the above information into a structured prompt template to ensure that the model can clearly understand and execute the task.

The final generated prompt is then utilized to invoke the large language model. Once the model has produced its output, additional processing of the returned data is conducted to ensure both the accuracy of the content and the correctness of the format.

The final output format is: *Case ID@*;*@*;*@*;*@Clinical Insights: ****. Dialectical Result: ****.*

4   Experiments

4.1   Dataset and Evaluation Metrics

The evaluation dataset consists of 300 medical case records collected and processed by the organizing team and stored in a self-built database. The TCM dialectical diagnosis questions are categorized into four types: clinical information, disease mechanism, syndrome, and explanation and summary, as illustrated in Fig. 5. The data is divided into training, leaderboard A, and leaderboard B sets in a ratio of 200:50:50, totaling 300 entries. The dataset is formatted in JSON.

{
    "Case Number": "Case 30",
    "Clinical Data": "Wang, male, 38 years old. First consultation: September 12, 1979. Chief complaint and medical history: Nosebleed for 15 days. On August 17, sudden nosebleed, with the most severe day having five episodes, each around 100-300ml, subsequently intermittent, accompanied by dizziness, thirst and dry nose, chest oppression and qi inversion, and dry stool. Examination: Pulse floating, large, and rapid at 84 beats/min, thin white tongue coating, red tongue body.",
    "Information Extraction Skill - Core Clinical Information": "Nosebleed; thirst and dry nose; chest oppression and qi inversion; dry stool; pulse floating, large and rapid",
    "Reasoning Ability - Pathogenesis Inference": "Nosebleed: Blood Heat Not Stable; Thirst and dry nose: Heat Injures Lung Collaterals; Dry stool: Heat Injures Lung Collaterals; Chest oppression and qi inversion: Heat Injures Lung Collaterals; Pulse floating, large and rapid: Heat Injures Lung Collaterals",
    "Information Extraction Skill - Core Pathogenesis": "Heat Injures Lung Collaterals; Blood Heat Not Stable",
    "Pathogenesis Answer": "H;J",
    "Pathogenesis Options": "A: Liver Stagnation; B: Injury to Yin and Qi Consumption; C: Dampness Obstruction; D: Yin Deficiency and Yang Hyperactivity; E: Damage to Heart Spirit; F: Injury to Central Qi; G: Disturbance of Spirit; H: Blood Heat Not Stable; I: Fluid Retention; J: Heat Injures Lung Collaterals",
    "Reasoning Ability - Syndrome Inference": "Heat Injures Lung Collaterals: Heat Injures Yang Collaterals; Blood Heat Not Stable: Reckless Movement of Blood Heat",
    "Information Extraction Skill - Core Syndrome": "Heat Injures Yang Collaterals; Reckless Movement of Blood Heat",
    "Syndrome Answer": "B;I",
    "Syndrome Options": "A: Disharmony of Spleen and Stomach; B: Reckless Movement of Blood Heat; C: Deficiency of Both Heart and Kidney; D: Damp-Heat Interaction; E: Evil Invading Pericardium; F: Wind Stirred by Summer Heat; G: Deficiency of Spleen and Kidney Yang; H: Phlegm Clouding the Orifices of the Heart; I: Heat Injures Yang Collaterals; J: Phlegm-Damp Internally Generated",
    "Clinical Experience": "Clinical experience: The patient was healthy prior to the sudden onset of nosebleeds. Given the rapid onset and the volume of the bleeding, it is indeed due to Heat Injures Lung Collaterals and Blood Heat Not Stable.",
    "Syndrome Differentiation": "Syndrome Differentiation: Heat Injures Yang Collaterals, Reckless Movement of Blood Heat"
}

Fig. 5. Data Sample.

Evaluation Metrics: The scoring criteria for each sub-task are detailed in Table 2. Given the varying significance of different tasks within the dialectical process, the weight distribution is set as follows. Syndrome: Disease Mechanism: Clinical Information: Explanation and Summary = 4:3:2:1. Consequently, the formula for calculating the total score is:

$$P = \frac{\sum(w_i * P_i)}{\sum(w_i)} \tag{1}$$

4.2   Experimental Setup

In this evaluation, we employed demonstration-guided and retrieval-augmented methods to direct the LLM in predicting answers for the test set without tuning

Table 2. Evaluation Metrics for TCM Diagnostic Thinking Skills.

Task	Evaluation Metric	Weight	Calculation	Score Range
Sub-task 1	Accuracy of identification and extraction (P1)	20%	P1 = Number of correct answers selected by model / Total correct answers	0-1
Sub-task 2	Accuracy of pathogenesis extraction (P2)	30%	P2 = Question score × Number of correct answers selected by model / (Total correct answers + Number of incorrect answers selected by model)	0-1
Sub-task 3	Accuracy of syndrome extraction (P3)	40%	P3 = Question score × Number of correct answers selected by model / (Total correct answers + Number of incorrect answers selected by model)	0-1
Sub-task 4	Overall quality of response (P4)	10%	P4 = Rouge-L	0-1
Task	Final Score (P)	100%	P = 0.2 × P1 + 0.3 × P2 + 0.4 × P3 + 0.1 × Rouge-L	0-1

any parameters. Specifically, we chose Qwen-Plus as the base model for task prediction and utilized bge-base-zh-v1.5 as the semantic retrieval model to fetch pertinent demonstrations from the training set. For the inference process, we configured the number of task examples to 2 and the number of retrieval-augmented knowledge examples to 1. The experiments were conducted on a Windows operating system, with Python 3.9.19 and the transformers library version 4.44.2.

4.3 Results and Analysis

We conducted comparative experiments on the TCM dialectical dataset, and Table 3 presents the performance of our method across all sub-tasks of the test set. It is important to note that, as the competition is still ongoing, we do not yet have access to the standard answers for the test set. Therefore, the results presented in this section are preliminary and derived from our ongoing experimentation.

First, we tested the Original Prompting method on Qwen-Plus by inputting all four tasks simultaneously into the model, resulting in a relatively low score of 22.73. By refining the prompt and integrating the TCM dialectical thinking chain, we achieved a significant improvement of 3.28 points, raising the score from 22.73 to 26.01. This demonstrates that incorporating the chain-of-thought

Table 3. Scores on different sub-tasks, with a final total score of 36.0.

Models	Task1	Task2	Task3	Task4	Total
Original Prompting	8.31	–	–	–	22.73
Prompting with CoT	8.46	–	–	–	26.01
+ Similar Demonstrations	–	–	–	–	28.73
+ Option Knowledge	–	–	–	–	30.39
+ Experiential Knowledge	–	–	16.69	–	36.00

enhances the model's performance and aligns well with the TCM dialectical thinking process.

Next, we verified that demonstration similarity positively impacts contextual learning. By comparing the results of similarity-based selection with those of random selection, we observed a substantial improvement of 2.72 points. This indicates that selecting demonstrations based on similarity is highly effective.

Finally, we further integrated the option knowledge enhancement and knowledge retrieval augmentation modules, which brought additional improvements of 1.66 and 5.61 points, respectively. Particularly, the knowledge retrieval augmentation module, which incorporates historical expert experience, contributed significantly to the improvement. This enhancement was particularly effective because it provided more precise training data, effectively addressing the issue of limited training data (only 200 entries in the training set, with content and distribution largely inconsistent with the test set).

In summary, our method demonstrated strong performance on the test set, achieving an overall score of 36.0 and placing among the top three participants. By introducing the TCM dialectical thinking chain, optimizing demonstration selection strategies, and enhancing option knowledge and knowledge retrieval, we significantly improved the model's reasoning ability and accuracy. These enhancements not only boosted the model's performance but also provided robust support for automating TCM dialectical thinking tasks.

5   Conclusion

This paper proposes a TCM dialectical framework that integrates chain-of-thought and retrieval augmentation. First, we introduced the TCM dialectical thinking chain, breaking down the task into clinical information extraction, disease mechanism inference, and syndrome diagnosis. Next, we scored all demonstrations in the candidate set and combined them according to their scores, filling them into the prompt template in a specific order. Finally, we introduced option knowledge enhancement and knowledge retrieval augmentation, which significantly improved the model's reasoning ability and accuracy. Through our proposed method, we achieved satisfactory results in this evaluation task.

Despite these achievements, we believe there is still considerable room for improvement. Firstly, fine-tuning the model with more specialized medical data could yield even better results for this task. Secondly, further exploration is needed in the construction of input templates. Constructing appropriate input templates for different tasks is crucial for accurately predicting the final answers.

References

1. Cheung, F.: Tcm: made in China. Nature **480**(7378), S82–S83 (2011)
2. Zong, H., et al.: Advancing Chinese biomedical text mining with community challenges. J. Biomed. Inf. **157**, 104716 (2024)

3. Hendrycks, D., et al.: Measuring massive multitask language understanding. arXiv preprint arXiv:2009.03300 (2020)
4. Huang, Y., et al.: C-eval: a multi-level multi-discipline Chinese evaluation suite for foundation models. Adv. Neural Inf. Process. Syst. **36** (2024)
5. Touvron, H., et al.: Llama: open and efficient foundation language models. arXiv preprint arXiv:2302.13971 (2023)
6. Taori, R., et al.: Stanford alpaca: an instruction-following llama model (2023)
7. Zhang, Z., Zhang, A., Li, M., Smola, A.: Automatic chain of thought prompting in large language models. arXiv preprint arXiv:2210.03493 (2022)
8. Wang, B., et al.: Towards understanding chain-of-thought prompting: an empirical study of what matters. arXiv preprint arXiv:2212.10001 (2022)
9. Chu, Z., et al.: A survey of chain of thought reasoning: advances. Front. Fut. (2023)
10. Ji, Z., et al.: Survey of hallucination in natural language generation. ACM Comput. Surv. **55**(12), 1–38 (2023)
11. Zhang, Y., et al.: Siren's song in the ai ocean: a survey on hallucination in large language models (2023). https://arxiv.org/abs/2309.01219
12. Chern, I., et al.: Factool: factuality detection in generative ai–a tool augmented framework for multi-task and multi-domain scenarios. arXiv preprint arXiv:2307.13528 (2023)
13. Huang, L., et al.: A survey on hallucination in large language models: principles, taxonomy, challenges, and open questions. arXiv preprint arXiv:2311.05232 (2023)
14. Ye, H., Liu, T., Zhang, A., Hua, W., Jia, W.: Cognitive mirage: a review of hallucinations in large language models. arXiv preprint arXiv:2309.06794 (2023)
15. Varshney, N., Yao, W., Zhang, H., Chen, J., Yu, D.: A stitch in time saves nine: detecting and mitigating hallucinations of llms by validating low-confidence generation. arXiv preprint arXiv:2307.03987 (2023)
16. Floridi, L., Chiriatti, M.: Gpt-3: its nature, scope, limits, and consequences. Mind. Mach. **30**, 681–694 (2020)
17. Anil, R., et al.: Palm 2 technical report. arXiv preprint arXiv:2305.10403 (2023)
18. Taylor, R., et al.: Galactica: a large language model for science. arXiv preprint arXiv:2211.09085 (2022)
19. Dubey, A., et al.: The llama 3 herd of models. arXiv preprint arXiv:2407.21783 (2024)
20. Zhao, W.X., et al.: A survey of large language models. arXiv preprint arXiv:2303.18223 (2023)
21. Brown, T.B.: Language models are few-shot learners. arXiv preprint arXiv:2005.14165 (2020)
22. Wei, J., et al.: Chain-of-thought prompting elicits reasoning in large language models. Adv. Neural Inf. Process. Syst. **35**, 24824–24837 (2022)
23. Hua, R., et al.: Lingdan: enhancing encoding of traditional Chinese medicine knowledge for clinical reasoning tasks with large language models. J. Am. Med. Inf. Assoc. **31**(9), 2019–2029 (2024)
24. Cai, Y., et al.: Medbench: a large-scale Chinese benchmark for evaluating medical large language models. In: Proceedings of the AAAI Conference on Artificial Intelligence, vol. 38, pp. 17709–17717 (2024)
25. Fan, W., et al.: A survey on rag meeting llms: towards retrieval-augmented large language models. In: Proceedings of the 30th ACM SIGKDD Conference on Knowledge Discovery and Data Mining, pp. 6491–6501 (2024)
26. Pham, P., Nguyen, L., Pedrycz, W., Vo, B.: Deep learning, graph-based text representation and classification: a survey, perspectives and challenges. Artif. Intell. Rev. **56**(6), 4893–4927 (2023)

Fine-Tuning Large Language Models for Syndrome Differentiation in Traditional Chinese Medicine

Wenlong Song[1], Zixuan Li[1], Huaiyu Wang[2], and Chi Yuan[1]([⊠])

[1] College of Computer Science and Software Engineering, Hohai University, Nanjing, China
20210021@hhu.edu.cn
[2] National Institute of Traditional Chinese Medicine Constitution and Preventive Treatment of Diseases, Beijing University of Chinese Medicine, Beijing, China

Abstract.

Objective: This study aims to enhance large language models (LLMs) performance on the TCMSD benchmark and strengthen their ability in Traditional Chinese Medicine (TCM) syndrome differentiation. The study explores the use of LLMs to model the complex reasoning processes inherent in TCM diagnosis.

Methods: We employed Quantized Low-Rank Adaptation (QLoRA) to fine-tune the Qwen2.5-72B model, specifically tailored to enhance its reasoning ability for TCM syndrome differentiation tasks. Additionally, ensemble learning techniques were utilized to further optimize model performance.

Results: Our method achieved a significant improvement on the TCMSD benchmark, reaching a performance score of 31.9050 with the Qwen2.5-72B + QLoRA + Ensemble method. Compared to the baseline Qwen2.5-7B, which scored 24.4804, our method resulted in an improvement of approximately 30.5%.

Conclusion: The results suggest that QLoRA fine-tuning, in combination with ensemble learning, can enhance the performance of LLMs in the context of TCM syndrome differentiation. This approach demonstrates the potential of leveraging advanced AI techniques to aid in the science of TCM, offering new opportunities for improving diagnostic accuracy and decision-making in clinical practice.

1 Introduction

Traditional Chinese Medicine (TCM) is a cornerstone of Chinese civilization, embodying profound wisdom and making significant contributions to public health [1]. Despite its long history and extensive application, the scientific principles underlying TCM remain challenging to articulate in a clear and accessible manner [2]. This difficulty poses a substantial barrier to the modernization and wider acceptance of TCM, necessitating innovative approaches to bridge the gap between traditional practices and contemporary scientific understanding.

© The Author(s), under exclusive license to Springer Nature Singapore Pte Ltd. 2025
Y. Zhang et al. (Eds.): CHIP 2024, CCIS 2458, pp. 39–52, 2025.
https://doi.org/10.1007/978-981-96-4298-4_4

In recent years, the rapid advancement of Artificial General Intelligence (AGI) has led to the emergence of large language models (LLMs) such as ChatGPT [3] and GLM-130B [4], which have demonstrated remarkable performance in natural language processing (NLP) tasks. These pretrained models possess the capability to process and comprehend vast amounts of data, uncovering latent knowledge and patterns that can be harnessed for various applications. LLMs enable the simulation of complex reasoning processes in TCM, enhancing syndrome differentiation and bridging traditional practices with modern scientific approaches for improved diagnostic accuracy and clinical decision-making [5].

A critical aspect of TCM is its syndrome differentiation thinking, which serves as the core methodology for diagnosis and treatment. This approach integrates clinical observations, theoretical knowledge, and practical experience, reflecting the unique characteristics and strengths of TCM [6]. By developing language models that incorporate syndrome differentiation thinking, it is possible to simulate the clinical reasoning processes of TCM practitioners [7]. Such models can provide interpretable analyses and support clinical decision-making, thereby facilitating the clear and effective communication of TCM's scientific principles. This integration of AI with TCM has the potential to overcome longstanding challenges, breaking down barriers between traditional medicine and modern technology, and laying the foundation for the modernization and internationalization of TCM [8]. Furthermore, recent explorations into AI comprehension of TCM knowledge, such as ChatGPT's understanding, are helping to enhance the fusion of traditional practices with advanced computational tools [9].

However, evaluating the diagnostic capabilities of LLMs in the context of TCM remains a significant challenge. Existing evaluation datasets, such as TCMBench [10] and Qibo-Benchmark [11], primarily assess basic TCM knowledge and lack the complexity required to evaluate comprehensive diagnostic reasoning. TCM diagnosis involves intricate processes of identification, judgment, and inference, which are not adequately captured by current benchmarks. This limitation hinders the ability to systematically and objectively assess the syndrome differentiation capabilities of language models, thereby restricting the optimization and improvement of LLMs within the TCM domain.

In this study, we focus on advancing the diagnostic reasoning capabilities of LLMs within the domain of TCM. By leveraging the TCM Syndrome Differentiation benchmark (TCMSD benchmark) provided by the 2024 CHIP Conference[1], we evaluate the ability of LLMs to perform syndrome differentiation, a core aspect of TCM diagnosis. Through fine-tuning the Qwen2.5-72B-Instruct model with Quantized Low-Rank Adaptation (QLoRA), we aim to address the complex reasoning processes inherent in TCM diagnostics. Furthermore, we integrate ensemble learning techniques to optimize the model's performance on the clinical information extraction task.

---

[1] http://cips-chip.org.cn/2024/eval1.

2   Related Work

2.1   Applications of Large Language Models in Medical Diagnosis

In recent years, LLMs have demonstrated significant potential in transforming medical diagnosis by leveraging their ability to process and analyze vast amounts of textual data. Models such as GPT-4 [12] have showcased their ability to assist in clinical decision-making, patient management, and medical literature synthesis [13]. Additionally, specialized models like BioGPT [14] and Radiology-LLama2 [15] have been fine-tuned for specific medical domains, achieving state-of-the-art performance in tasks such as biomedical text generation and radiology interpretation. Notably, fine-tuned LLMs have also made significant strides in medical question answering [16] and clinical text de-identification [17]. Furthermore, the development of open-source pretrained models such as Biomistral [18] has broadened access to powerful medical LLMs for researchers and healthcare professionals. Biomedical text mining has further been advanced by community challenge evaluation competitions, which play a crucial role in fostering innovation and collaboration [19]. However, despite these advancements, challenges remain in integrating domain-specific knowledge, ensuring explainability, and addressing ethical considerations in medical applications [20].

2.2   Development of Large Language Models in Traditional Chinese Medicine

The application of LLMs in the field of TCM is an emerging area of research [5]. Unlike Western medicine, TCM emphasizes holistic diagnosis based on syndrome differentiation, a reasoning process that integrates symptoms, pulse patterns, and historical context. Existing LLMs often struggle to model these intricate relationships due to the unique terminologies, diagnostic principles, and cultural nuances inherent to TCM [9].

To address this gap, recent studies have explored the use of LLMs tailored for TCM-specific tasks, such as Qibo [11], Lingdan [21], TCMChat [22], TCM-GPT [23], BianCang [24]. Despite these advancements, the complexity of TCM reasoning continues to pose significant challenges for LLMs, such as the need for interpretability and the alignment of model outputs with traditional diagnostic frameworks.

A critical aspect of TCM practice is syndrome differentiation, which serves as the core methodology for diagnosis and treatment. It reflects the essence of TCM itself, where diagnosis is not based solely on isolated symptoms but rather on the interconnections between multiple factors.

2.3   Low-Rank Adaptation and Ensemble Learning

Low-Rank Adaptation (LoRA) [25] has emerged as a leading paradigm in parameter-efficient fine-tuning, enabling the adaptation of dense neural networks by introducing pluggable low-rank matrices. By decomposing weight updates into low-rank matrices, LoRA significantly reduces the number of trainable parameters while maintaining or even improving task performance. Recent studies have demonstrated the efficacy of LoRA across various domains. For example, Hu et al. [26] proposed QLoRA, a method for fine-tuning quantized LLMs that retains high performance while minimizing resource requirements. This technique has been extended to specialized tasks, such as sentiment analysis [27] and machine translation [28], showcasing LoRA's versatility in adapting to diverse applications. Moreover, LoRA has shown promise in domain-specific contexts, such as medical diagnosis, where fine-tuned LLMs assist in generating accurate and context-aware diagnoses [29]. These advancements highlight LoRA's ability to balance efficiency and effectiveness, making it a cornerstone of modern machine learning practices.

Ensemble learning, on the other hand, focuses on improving model performance and robustness by combining the predictions of multiple models or learning algorithms [30]. In recent years, ensemble learning has seen significant advancements, particularly in the development of efficient and robust algorithms. Modern boosting techniques, such as Gradient Boosting Machines, XGBoost [31], LightGBM [32], and CatBoost [33], have improved computational efficiency and handling of complex data structures, making them highly popular in both academic research and industry applications. Additionally, the integration of ensemble methods with deep learning, such as Deep Ensembles [34], has enabled better uncertainty estimation and robustness in neural networks, paving the way for more reliable predictions in safety-critical applications.

This study focus on the syndrome differentiation task, fine-tuning the Qwen2.5-72B-Instruct model using Quantized Low-Rank Adaptation (QLoRA). Our goal is to enhance the model's performance in these tasks, thereby advancing the use of LLMs in TCM diagnostics. By leveraging the TCMSD benchmark provided by the 2024 CHIP Conference, we aim to systematically evaluate the capabilities and limitations of LLMs in the context of TCM syndrome differentiation, offering insights into their potential applications in this unique domain.

3 Methods

In this study, we aim to enhance both the performance of LLMs in TCM syndrome differentiation and the interpretability of the syndrome differentiation process in TCM. To achieve this, we combine two key methodologies: QLoRA for efficient fine-tuning and ensemble learning for enhanced clinical information extraction. We use the Qwen 2.5-72B-Instruct model as the base model, fine-tuning it on the TCMSD benchmark, a specialized dataset designed to evaluate diagnostic reasoning in TCM. QLoRA enables the fine-tuning of LLMs with reduced memory and computational costs, while ensemble learning enhances the accuracy and robustness of the model by combining predictions from multiple training rounds.

3.1   TCMSD Benchmark

The TCMSD benchmark is a specialized evaluation framework developed to assess the diagnostic reasoning capabilities of LLMs in TCM, with a primary focus on syndrome differentiation. It is based on the structured reasoning process inherent to TCM diagnostic practices, encompassing four key tasks: Clinical Information Extraction, Pathogenesis Inference, Syndrome Inference, and Diagnostic Summarization.

The benchmark dataset consists of 300 curated clinical cases, divided into training, validation, and test sets in a 200:50:50 ratio. These cases were manually curated to reflect the diagnostic reasoning process of TCM practitioners, ensuring high quality and relevance.

The TCMSD benchmark provides a quantifiable and standardized method for evaluating LLM performance in complex TCM reasoning scenarios. It supports the development of models capable of both accurate syndrome differentiation and effective interpretation of diagnostic reasoning in TCM.

Dataset Description. The TCMSD benchmark dataset is structured to comprehensively capture the critical components of TCM diagnostic reasoning. Each clinical case in the dataset is annotated with attributes that allow the evaluation of various tasks such as clinical information extraction, pathogenesis inference, syndrome inference, and diagnostic summarization. The primary attributes in the dataset are as follows:

- **Clinical Information:** Foundational patient data, including chief complaints, medical history, physical examination findings, and laboratory results. This information forms the basis for the diagnostic reasoning process. For example, "王某，男，38岁。初诊:1979年9月12日。主诉及病史:鼻流血15天。8月17日，突然鼻流血，最严重的一天流血5次，每次约100 300ml，继而时出时止，头昏晕痛，口渴鼻干，胸闷气逆，大便干。诊查:脉浮大数、84次/分，舌苔薄白、舌质红。" (Example: Mr. Wang, male, 38 years old. First visit: September 12, 1979. Chief complaint and history: nasal bleeding for 15 days...)

- **Information Extraction Ability - Key Clinical Information:** Extracted clinical information that is essential for pathogenesis inference, such as specific symptoms, signs, and other relevant data points. For example, "鼻流血;口渴鼻干;胸闷气逆;大便干;脉浮大数" (Key clinical information: nasal bleeding; dry mouth and nose; chest tightness with counterflow; dry stools; floating, large, rapid pulse).

- **Information Extraction Ability - Key Pathogenesis:** Core pathogenesis inferred from the clinical data. For example, "热伤肺络;血热不固" (Key pathogenesis: heat injuring lung collaterals; blood heat failing to retain).

- **Inference Ability - Pathogenesis Inference:** The inferred pathogenesis derived from the extracted clinical information. This step aligns with TCM's theoretical approach to disease causation. For example, "鼻流血:血热不固;口渴鼻干:热伤肺络;大便干:热伤肺络;胸闷气逆:热伤肺络;脉浮大数:热伤肺络"

(Pathogenesis inference: nasal bleeding - blood heat failing to retain; dry mouth and nose - heat injuring lung collaterals...).

- **Pathogenesis Options:** Multiple-choice options for pathogenesis, from which the model must choose appropriate answer(s). For example, "A:肝郁; B:伤阴耗气; C:湿邪阻滞... H:血热不固; I:水饮内停; J:热伤肺络" (Options: A: Liver constraint; B: Yin injury and Qi depletion; C: Damp obstruction... H: Blood heat failing to retain; I: Water retention; J: Heat injuring lung collaterals).
- **Pathogenesis Answer:** The correct reference answer(s) for pathogenesis, serving as the standard for evaluating the model's inference capabilities. For example, "H; J".
- **Inference Ability - Syndrome Inference:** The model's inferred syndrome diagnosis, which represents the final diagnostic result in TCM based on the identified pathogenesis. For example, "热伤肺络:热伤阳络;血热不固:血热妄行" (Syndrome inference: heat injuring lung collaterals - heat injuring yang collaterals; blood heat failing to retain - reckless movement of blood heat).
- **Information Extraction Ability - Key Syndrome:** Key syndrome components derived from the pathogenesis, used to assess the model's understanding of TCM syndrome differentiation. For example, "热伤阳络;血热妄行" (Key syndrome: heat injuring yang collaterals; reckless movement of blood heat).
- **Syndrome Answer:** The correct answer(s) for syndrome diagnosis, used as a reference for evaluating the model's output. For example, "B; I".
- **Syndrome Options:** Multiple-choice options for syndrome diagnosis, from which the model selects the correct syndrome. Each option represents a potential TCM syndrome. For example, "A:脾胃不和; B:血热妄行; C:心肾两亏... I:热伤阳络; J:痰湿内蕴" (Options: A: Spleen-stomach disharmony; B: Reckless movement of blood heat; C: Heart-kidney deficiency... I: Heat injuring yang collaterals; J: Phlegm-damp retention).
- **Clinical Insights:** Interpretive insights derived during the diagnostic process, offering contextual understanding of the model's reasoning. For example, "患者素体健康，今突发鼻衄，观其来势之迅猛，衄血量之多，实系热伤肺络、血热不固。" (Clinical insights: The patient was generally healthy, but now has sudden onset of nasal bleeding. Given its rapid onset and large volume, it is a case of heat injuring lung collaterals and blood heat failing to retain).
- **Syndrome Differentiation:** The final result of syndrome differentiation, representing the model's ultimate diagnostic conclusion. For example, "热伤阳络，血热妄行" (Syndrome differentiation: Heat injuring yang collaterals, reckless movement of blood heat).

3.2 Task Description

The task is organized to formalize the syndrome differentiation process in TCM which can be broken down into four key steps (Fig. 1):

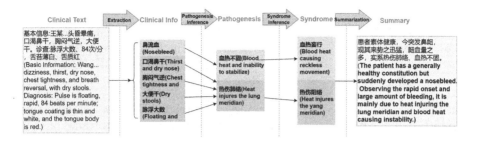

Fig. 1. Task Description

1. **Clinical Information Extraction:** This step involves extracting clinical information from case text, including general symptoms and signs, tongue and pulse diagnosis, etiological factors, and test results.
2. **Pathogenesis Inference:** Using the extracted clinical information, the underlying pathogenesis is inferred and determined.
3. **Syndrome Inference:** Based on the inferred pathogenesis, the final diagnostic conclusion, known as the syndrome, is made.
4. **Diagnostic summarization:** This step synthesizes the previous steps, providing an explanation and summary of the diagnostic reasoning process. This includes clinical insights and the final diagnostic results.

3.3 Evaluation Metrics

The TCMSD benchmark utilizes a comprehensive evaluation framework to assess the model's performance across four key sub-tasks: Clinical Information Extraction, Pathogenesis Inference, Syndrome Inference, and Diagnostic Summarization. Each sub-task contributes a weighted score to the overall evaluation metric P. The metrics are defined as follows:

– **P1**
  This metric evaluates the accuracy of the model in extracting relevant clinical information from the input data. It is calculated as:

$$P_1 = \frac{\text{Number of extracted correct data points}}{\text{Total number of correct data points in the answer}} \quad (1)$$

– **P2**
  This metric measures the model's ability to infer the underlying pathogenesis based on the extracted clinical information. It is calculated as:

$$P_2 = \frac{\text{Number of correct answers selected by the model}}{\text{Total number of correct answers} + \text{Number of incorrect answers}} \quad (2)$$

– **P3**
  This metric evaluates the precision and accuracy of the model in deducing the correct syndrome from the inferred pathogenesis. It is defined as:

$$P_3 = \frac{\text{Number of correct answers selected by the model}}{\text{Total number of correct answers} + \text{Number of incorrect answers}} \quad (3)$$

- **P4**

This metric assesses the overall quality of the model's explanatory responses by comparing them to reference answers using the Rouge-L score:

$$P_4 = \text{Rouge-L score} \tag{4}$$

The final performance score P is calculated as a weighted sum of the individual sub-task scores, with weights assigned based on the relative importance of each task in diagnostic reasoning:

$$P = 0.2 \times P_1 + 0.3 \times P_2 + 0.4 \times P_3 + 0.1 \times P_4 \tag{5}$$

This weighting scheme reflects the significance of complex reasoning tasks such as syndrome inference (highest weight) and balances it with the importance of accurate extraction, inference, and response quality.

3.4   QLoRA Fine-Tuning

QLoRA is an efficient approach for fine-tuning large pretrained models, particularly in resource-constrained environments. It leverages two key techniques: quantization and low-rank matrix decomposition [25].

Quantization: QLoRA applies quantization to reduce the precision of model weights, significantly decreasing memory and computational requirements. In our experiments, we utilize 4-bit quantization, which reduces the model size without sacrificing performance. To further optimize memory usage, we employ double quantization, which adds an extra layer of quantization to the quantization constants. The first layer reduces the precision of the model weights, while the second layer compresses the metadata (e.g., scale and zero-point values) using a similar approach. This dual-layer strategy minimizes the storage requirements for quantization parameters, allowing larger models to fit into limited hardware resources. The combination of 4-bit quantization and double quantization results in substantial memory savings while maintaining high accuracy in syndrome differentiation tasks. By managing the model's memory footprint effectively, large models such as Qwen2.5:72B can be fine-tuned on two 48GB GPUs and deployed on a single GPU, enhancing their applicability in real-world TCM scenarios.

Low-Rank Adaptation: Instead of fine-tuning the entire model, QLoRA introduces low-rank matrices to adapt specific layers of the model to the target task. Specifically, we focus on the attention mechanism, which involves the query (Q), key (K), value (V), and output (O) matrices, central to capturing contextual relationships in transformer-based models.

Each matrix is decomposed into a low-rank approximation, significantly reducing the number of parameters that need to be updated during fine-tuning. This allows us to adapt only the relevant parameters associated with the attention mechanism, while leaving the majority of the model's parameters unchanged. As a result, memory usage and computational costs are reduced, making the adaptation process more efficient.

3.5 Ensemble Learning for Clinical Information Extraction

To improve the robustness and accuracy of clinical information extraction for TCM syndrome differentiation, we employ ensemble learning, combining models trained over different training rounds. This approach leverages the complementary strengths of models at various stages of training to enhance the overall performance of the extraction task.

Let $M_1, M_2, \ldots, M_n$ represent the models trained in different rounds. For each case, the extracted clinical information is defined as:

$$E = \bigcup_{i=1}^{n} E_{M_i} \tag{6}$$

where E_{M_i} denotes the set of clinical information extracted by model M_i.

Example: Assume we train three models (M_1, M_2, M_3), each with different training rounds. The extracted clinical information sets are as follows:

- $E_{M_1} = \{$fatigue, pale complexion, weak pulse$\}$
- $E_{M_2} = \{$dizziness, weak pulse$\}$
- $E_{M_3} = \{$fatigue, pale complexion, dizziness$\}$

The ensemble prediction, obtained by taking the union of these sets, is:

$$E = E_{M_1} \cup E_{M_2} \cup E_{M_3} = \{\text{fatigue, pale complexion, dizziness, weak pulse}\} \tag{7}$$

The union of predictions broadens the coverage of extracted information, improving the model's ability to identify relevant clinical details comprehensively.

4 Evaluation

4.1 Hyperparameter Settings

The hyperparameters used in our fine-tuning experiments were selected through multiple rounds of experimentation to optimize the performance on the TCM syndrome differentiation task. The final set of hyperparameters, determined based on empirical results, is detailed in Table 1.

These hyperparameters were chosen after extensive experimentation to ensure both efficient training and high accuracy in the TCM syndrome differentiation task.

Table 1. Hyperparameters for Fine-Tuning.

Hyperparameter	Value
Learning Rate	4×10^{-3} (linear decay)
Batch Size	8
Optimizer	AdamW [35]
Weight Decay	0.01
Low-Rank Decomposition Rank	16 (for Q, K, V, and O matrices)
Training Duration	4 epochs, 4 h on two NVIDIA A6000 GPUs

4.2   Results

This experiment evaluates the performance of Qwen2.5 models with varying parameter sizes (7B to 72B), using different reasoning methods (Step-by-Step vs. End-to-End), and incorporating advanced techniques like QLoRA and ensemble learning.

Table 2. Ablation results for Qwen2.5-7B models with different methods. Note: (s) indicates Step-by-Step reasoning, while (e) indicates End-to-End reasoning.

Method	P1	P2	P3	P4	P
7B(s)	6.8843	5.0799	8.2371	0.9596	21.1609
7B(e)	6.7555	5.2345	11.2428	1.2476	24.4804
7B(e) + QLoRA	6.8375	6.5724	12.7426	1.3278	27.4803
7B(e) + QLoRA + Ensemble	7.3525	6.5724	12.7426	1.3278	27.9953
14B(s)	6.7869	5.2417	8.9920	1.1722	22.1928
14B(e)	7.2204	5.9442	11.1243	1.1499	25.4388
14B(e) + QLoRA	6.5987	6.9251	13.4144	1.5211	28.4593
14B(e) + QLoRA + Ensemble	6.9793	6.9251	13.4144	1.5211	28.8399
32B(s)	6.5526	6.7720	10.3763	1.1333	24.8342
32B(e)	7.1120	6.5255	12.0029	1.3927	27.0331
32B(e) + QLoRA	7.8296	7.5182	13.2271	1.4617	30.0366
32B(e) + QLoRA + Ensemble	7.8864	7.5182	13.2271	1.4617	30.0934
72B(s)	7.2247	6.5540	10.7333	1.3438	25.8558
72B(e)	7.2009	6.6746	12.1713	**1.5474**	27.5942
72B(e) + QLoRA	7.7712	7.7899	14.7000	1.4438	31.7050
72B(e) + QLoRA + Ensemble	**7.9712**	**7.7899**	**14.7000**	1.4438	**31.9050**

Building on the observations from Table 2, a direct comparison between the 7B and 72B models highlights the substantial impact of model size on performance. Specifically, the 7B(e) model achieves a performance score of 24.4804, while the 72B(e) model reaches 27.5942, indicating a performance increase of 12.7%. This result underscores the benefit of scaling up model parameters, with the larger 72B model demonstrating better capability in handling TCM syndrome differentiation task. Furthermore, the 72B model, when combined with QLoRA and ensemble learning, achieves the highest performance across all metrics, with a final score of 31.9050, further emphasizing the synergistic effects of model size, fine-tuning, and ensemble techniques in enhancing accuracy and robustness.

5   Discussion

This study demonstrates the significant potential of advanced techniques like QLoRA fine-tuning and ensemble learning in improving the performance of LLMs for the complex task of TCM syndrome differentiation. Our results show that the combination of QLoRA and ensemble learning with the Qwen2.5-72B model led to a notable performance increase on the TCMSD benchmark, with an improvement of approximately 30.5% compared to the baseline Qwen2.5-7B model. Below, we discuss the strengths of our approach, and the limitations we encountered.

5.1   Strengths of the Approach

Two key strengths of our methodology contribute to its effectiveness:

- **Efficient Fine-Tuning:** QLoRA's ability to fine-tune large models with low-rank adaptation and quantization allows us to optimize the Qwen2.5-72B model for TCM syndrome differentiation while reducing computational and memory requirements. This makes fine-tuning large models more feasible in resource-constrained environments.
- **Interpretability:** The focus on TCM syndrome differentiation underscored the potential of LLMs to provide interpretable results, supporting clinical decision-making and enhancing understanding of TCM diagnostic processes.

5.2   Limitations

Despite the promising results, two limitations remain:

Limited TCM Knowledge in LLMs: While fine-tuning with QLoRA improved performance, pretrained LLMs still lack comprehensive domain-specific knowledge about TCM. This limits their ability to fully understand the complex concepts inherent in TCM diagnosis, suggesting that further domain adaptation is necessary. Potential solutions to address this limitation include:

- **Continuous Pretraining on TCM-Focused Corpora:** Incorporating more extensive, domain-specific knowledge by continuously pretraining the model on larger, TCM-focused datasets. This approach would help the model better understand the unique concepts, terminologies, and reasoning processes in TCM.
- **Hybrid Models Combining Expert Knowledge with LLMs:** Utilizing hybrid models that combine the strengths of LLMs with expert knowledge, such as rule-based systems or knowledge graphs, to enhance the model's diagnostic reasoning. These models can provide structure and consistency to the reasoning process in TCM.
- **Retrieval-Augmented Generation (RAG):** Implementing RAG methods, where the model dynamically retrieves relevant, up-to-date information from external TCM knowledge bases or resources during inference. This can provide the model with richer, context-specific knowledge that it may not have been trained on directly, improving performance and decision-making.

Dataset Limitations: The TCMSD benchmark dataset, though useful, is relatively small. This restricts the model's ability to generalize to the wide variety of real-world clinical scenarios encountered in TCM practice, necessitating further expansion of the dataset for more robust training and evaluation. To address this, an increased dataset size, including diverse clinical cases, or the application of data augmentation techniques, could enhance the model's generalization ability.

6   Conclusion

This study demonstrates that combining QLoRA fine-tuning and ensemble learning significantly enhances the diagnostic reasoning capabilities of LLMs in TCM syndrome differentiation. The findings underscore the potential of advanced AI techniques to modernize and internationalize TCM practices. Addressing current challenges and exploring future research directions can further optimize the integration of LLMs into TCM diagnostics, enabling innovative applications in clinical practice.

Acknowledgments. This study is supported by National Natural Science Foundation of China (62302151) and Fundamental Research Funds for the Central Universities (B220202076)

References

1. Wang, W.Y., Zhou, H., Wang, Y.F., Sang, B.S., Liu, L.: Current policies and measures on the development of traditional Chinese medicine in China. Pharmacol. Res. **163**, 105187 (2021)

2. Huang, N., Huang, W., Wu, J., Long, S., Luo, Y., Huang, J.: Possible opportunities and challenges for traditional Chinese medicine research in 2035. Front. Pharmacol. **15**, 1426300 (2024)
3. Kasneci, E., et al.: Chatgpt for good? on opportunities and challenges of large language models for education. Learn. Individ. Differ. **103**, 102274 (2023)
4. GLM, T., et al.: Chatglm: a family of large language models from glm-130b to glm-4 all tools. arXiv preprint arXiv:2406.12793 (2024)
5. Zijia, C., et al.: The application, challenges, and prospects of large language models in the field of traditional chinese medicine. Med. J. Peking Union Med. Coll. Hosp. (2024)
6. Tang, J.L., Liu, B.Y., Ma, K.W.: Traditional Chinese medicine. The Lancet **372**(9654), 1938–1940 (2008)
7. Matos, L.C., Machado, J.P., Monteiro, F.J., Greten, H.J.: Understanding traditional Chinese medicine therapeutics: an overview of the basics and clinical applications. In: Healthcare, vol. 9, p. 257. MDPI (2021)
8. Zhao, Z., et al.: Prevention and treatment of covid-19 using traditional Chinese medicine: a review. Phytomedicine **85**, 153308 (2021)
9. Yizhen, L., Shaohan, H., Jiaxing, Q., Lei, Q., Dongran, H., Zhongzhi, L.: Exploring the comprehension of chatgpt in traditional Chinese medicine knowledge. arXiv preprint arXiv:2403.09164 (2024)
10. Yue, W., et al.: Tcmbench: a comprehensive benchmark for evaluating large language models in traditional Chinese medicine. arXiv preprint arXiv:2406.01126 (2024)
11. Zhang, H., et al.: Qibo: a large language model for traditional Chinese medicine. arXiv preprint arXiv:2403.16056 (2024)
12. Achiam, J., et al.: Gpt-4 technical report. arXiv preprint arXiv:2303.08774 (2023)
13. Waisberg, E., et al.: Gpt-4: a new era of artificial intelligence in medicine. Irish J. Med. Sci. (1971-) **192**(6), 3197–3200 (2023)
14. Luo, R., et al.: Biogpt: generative pre-trained transformer for biomedical text generation and mining. Brief. Bioinf. **23**(6), bbac409 (2022)
15. Liu, Z., et al.: Radiology-llama2: best-in-class large language model for radiology. arXiv preprint arXiv:2309.06419 (2023)
16. Singhal, K., et al.: Towards expert-level medical question answering with large language models. arXiv preprint arXiv:2305.09617 (2023)
17. Liu, Z., et al.: Deid-gpt: zero-shot medical text de-identification by gpt-4. arXiv preprint arXiv:2303.11032 (2023)
18. Labrak, Y., Bazoge, A., Morin, E., Gourraud, P.A., Rouvier, M., Dufour, R.: Biomistral: a collection of open-source pretrained large language models for medical domains. arXiv preprint arXiv:2402.10373 (2024)
19. Zong, H., et al.: Advancing Chinese biomedical text mining with community challenges. J. Biomed. Inf., 104716 (2024)
20. Ullah, E., Parwani, A., Baig, M.M., Singh, R.: Challenges and barriers of using large language models (llm) such as chatgpt for diagnostic medicine with a focus on digital pathology-a recent scoping review. Diagn. Pathol. **19**(1), 43 (2024)
21. Hua, R., et al.: Lingdan: enhancing encoding of traditional Chinese medicine knowledge for clinical reasoning tasks with large language models. J. Am. Med. Inf. Assoc. **31**(9), 2019–2029 (2024)
22. Dai, Y., et al.: Tcmchat: a generative large language model for traditional Chinese medicine. Pharmacol. Res., 107530 (2024)

23. Yang, G., Liu, X., Shi, J., Wang, Z., Wang, G.: Tcm-gpt: efficient pre-training of large language models for domain adaptation in traditional Chinese medicine. Comput. Methods Prog. Biomed. Update, 100158 (2024)

24. Wei, S., et al.: Biancang: a traditional Chinese medicine large language model. arXiv preprint arXiv:2411.11027 (2024)

25. Hu, E.J., et al.: Lora: low-rank adaptation of large language models. arXiv preprint arXiv:2106.09685 (2021)

26. Hu, E.J., et al.: Qlora: efficient finetuning of quantized llms. arXiv preprint arXiv:2304.05439 (2023)

27. Liu, W., Zhang, H., Li, M.: Fine-tuning language models with qlora for sentiment analysis. J. Nat. Lang. Process. **30**, 123–135 (2023)

28. Zhang, L., Wang, Y., Chen, L.: Efficient machine translation with qlora. Mach. Transl. J. **45**, 456–470 (2023)

29. Chen, X., Liu, K., Zhang, W.: Medical diagnosis assistance using qlora-finetuned large language models. J. Med. Artif. Intell. **8**, 200–215 (2023)

30. Mienye, I.D., Sun, Y.: A survey of ensemble learning: concepts, algorithms, applications, and prospects. IEEE Access **10**, 99129–99149 (2022)

31. Chen, T., Guestrin, C.: Xgboost: a scalable tree boosting system. In: Proceedings of the 22nd ACM SIGKDD International Conference on Knowledge Discovery and Data Mining, pp. 785–794 (2016)

32. Ke, G., et al.: Lightgbm: a highly efficient gradient boosting decision tree. Adv. Neural Inf. Process. Syst. **30** (2017)

33. Prokhorenkova, L., Gusev, G., Vorobev, A., Dorogush, A.V., Gulin, A.: Catboost: unbiased boosting with categorical features. Adv. Neural Inf. Process. Syst. **31** (2018)

34. Lakshminarayanan, B., Pritzel, A., Blundell, C.: Simple and scalable predictive uncertainty estimation using deep ensembles. Adv. Neural Inf. Process. Syst. **30** (2017)

35. Loshchilov, I.: Decoupled weight decay regularization. arXiv preprint arXiv:1711.05101 (2017)

Iterative Retrieval Augmentation for Syndrome Differentiation via Large Language Models

Qiluo Chao[1]($\boxtimes$) (ID), Zeyu Zhang[1] (ID), Meng Zhan[2] (ID), and Xian Zhang[1] (ID)

[1] School of Information Engineering, Chang'an University, Xi'an, China
chaoql@126.com
[2] The First Affiliated Hospital of Anhui University of Chinese Medicine, Anhui University of Chinese Medicine, Hefei, China

Abstract. Traditional medical research is an important application scenario for natural language processing, and the differentiation of the Traditional Chinese Medicine (TCM) syndrome is an important challenge among them. We research the TCM syndrome differentiation process proposed in Evaluation 1 of the 10th China Conference on Health Information Processing (CHIP 2024) and propose a TCM syndrome differentiation method based on iterative retrieval-enhanced generation technology. A general large language model can achieve relatively high accuracy in a small-sample knowledge database. The method organically combines pathogenesis reasoning and syndrome reasoning, and the two work together to refine and improve the accuracy of syndrome differentiation. The experimental results on the test dataset show that the method proposed in this paper is effective, with a final score of 32.0534, ranking fifth in this task.

Keywords: Retrieval-augmented Generation · Chain-of-Thought prompting · Large Language Models

1 Introduction

With the success of large language models (LLMs) in natural language processing(NLP), medicine, an important application field of NLP, has received great attention in recent years [1]. Many studies have explored the combination of LLMs and medicine, including assisted diagnosis and treatment [2], medical imaging [3], health management [4], and drug development [5–7].

However, the scientific principles of TCM are difficult to present in an easy-to-understand way. As Syndrome Differentiation [8] is the core of traditional medical diagnosis and treatment, using artificial intelligence to realize automated TCM syndrome differentiation is an important challenge [9]. With the successive emergence of evaluation datasets in the field of TCM [10,11], many studies fine-tune general LLMs based on these datasets to achieve vertical-domain question

© The Author(s), under exclusive license to Springer Nature Singapore Pte Ltd. 2025
Y. Zhang et al. (Eds.): CHIP 2024, CCIS 2458, pp. 53–63, 2025.
https://doi.org/10.1007/978-981-96-4298-4_5

answering. However this technology has excessively high requirements for hardware equipment, and parameterized knowledge is difficult to update. Conducting Syndrome Differentiation research based on retrieval-enhanced generation technology seems to be a more efficient solution. Knowledge injection into LLMs can be completed by simply updating the knowledge base. However, how to achieve high-precision retrieval and improve the relevance between the retrieved TCM knowledge and the requirements is a problem.

The 10th China Health Information Processing Conference (CHIP 2024), with the theme "Large Models in Medical Vertical Domains", proposed three assessment tasks. Among them, Task 1 is the evaluation task for TCM syndrome differentiation. The use of LLMs is required to perform differentiation reasoning for the TCM syndrome based on existing TCM [12]theories. Using the given clinical data, let the model make a diagnosis through steps such as identification, reasoning, and judgment.

This paper studies the small sample dataset provided by the organizers and proposes an iterative retrieval-enhanced syndrome differentiation framework. Iterative retrieval technology (Iter-RAG) enables the LLM to utilize the generated output of the previous iteration to improve the query in each iteration, so as to retrieve relevant knowledge more precisely and thus improve the answer generation in the next iteration. Based on the existing dependency between pathogenesis and syndromes, the syndrome inference is collaboratively refined. Compared with the traditional single retrieval-enhanced method, it has improved by 36.60%. In the evaluation round A, it achieved a score of 30.3406.

2   Related Work

2.1   Large Language Models

Large language models (LLMs) such as GPT-3 [13], T5 [14], and LLaMA [15] typically contain hundreds of billions of parameters. After pre-training on large-scale mixed source corpora, they demonstrate powerful natural language understanding and generation capabilities. With the development of instruction fine-tuning [16] and benchmark testing [17], the applications of LLMs in the medical field are becoming more extensive and in-depth. By combining expert knowledge and real conversation data, LLMs can effectively handle complex medical conversations and provide professional advice [2,4]. Interdisciplinary cooperation is particularly important in the field of natural language processing. Vertical domain models in medicine can significantly improve the efficiency of drug research and development and predict drug efficacy [5–7]. As the first large-scale visual language model in the Chinese medical field, Qilin-Med-VL [3], after feature alignment and instruction tuning, performs outstandingly in generating medical image descriptions and answering complex medical questions.

2.2   Retrieval-Augmented Generation

Retrieval-Augmented Generation (RAG) [18] reduces hallucinations in LLMs generation through retrieval. Especially in professional knowledge fields such as TCM diagnosis, RAG can combine external knowledge base information with general LLMs to provide strong support for question answering. Some researchers retrieve real similar documents from the knowledge base by generating hypothesis documents related to queries [19] or changing the retrieval granularity [20]. Iter-RAG [21,22] can significantly improve factual accuracy [23] in complex multi-step reasoning tasks.

2.3 Chain-of-Thought Prompting

Chain-of-Thought (CoT) can guide LLM to generate intermediate reasoning steps of the final answer, thus enhancing the logical reasoning ability of LLM [24,25]. Research shows that Zero-Shot-CoT, which guides LLMs to think step by step [26], has achieved significant improvements in reasoning tasks. In the current challenge, we manually design the chain-of-thought steps to directionally guide the large model to complete reasoning by simulating the thinking mode of human doctors.

3   Task Analysis

The task is decomposed into four subtasks to guide the model to reason under the framework of syndrome differentiation thinking. The purpose is to test the model's understanding and execution ability of each link of the TCM syndrome differentiation process and ensure that it can accurately identify, infer and summarize core clinical information, so as to obtain complete syndrome differentiation results. Next, we will introduce these specific subtasks.

1. Core clinical information extraction. First, according to the description in the clinical data, identify and extract core clinical information, including "pale complexion", "white and greasy tongue and pulse", "fear", etc. Core clinical information is the first-hand data for syndrome differentiation, and complete and detailed data is helpful for subsequent pathomechanisms inference.
2. Pathomechanisms inference [27]. Infer the pathomechanisms based on the identified core clinical information. Possible pathomechanisms are provided in the options, such as "wind movement on fire", "a deficiency of qi and blood", "insomnia due to gallbladder deficiency", etc. Pathomechanisms inference needs to be combined with clinical data and refer to TCM theory to determine the possible pathogenesis mechanism, to further summarize it into specific syndromes.
3. Syndrome differentiation. Combine the pathomechanisms inferred in the previous step to obtain the final syndrome. The purpose of this step is to summarize the complete syndrome differentiation results and select from the selection types such as "a deficiency of qi in the heart and gallbladder" and "disharmony of the spleen and stomach". Syndrome differentiation is the process of inferring syndromes from pathomechanisms and finally forming a diagnosis.

4. Interpretation and summary. In the interpretation and summary, the above syndrome differentiation process is summarized to obtain clinical experience. The consultation part can be an analysis of the characteristics of the disease, and the syndrome differentiation result should be the final diagnosis, which will provide subsequent treatment guidance.

4 Methodology

4.1 Overview

In this section, the evaluated solutions will be introduced. As shown in Fig. 1, the solutions are divided into two parts: Data preprocessing and storage and subtask collaborative inference. Among them, the key to subtask collaborative inference lies in the Iterative Retrieval Augmentation Generation Process and Prompt Generation.

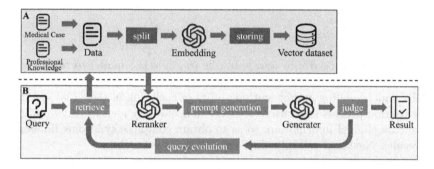

Fig. 1. The overview of our method. (A) Data preprocessing and storage. (B) The collaborative reasoning process of four sub-tasks.

4.2 Data Preprocessing and Storage

As shown in Fig. 2, the medical case data in JSON format, is divided into blocks according to objects and segmented into four sub-datasets corresponding to sub-tasks to facilitate subsequent retrieval for different tasks and one iterative dataset for sub-task 2. The professional knowledge data in TXT format, is cut according to a fixed length of 512 tokens. The overlapping length between two adjacent chunks is 20 tokens. The processed text blocks are embedded using the bge-large-zh-v1.5 model transformed into vectors and stored in the Qdrant database.

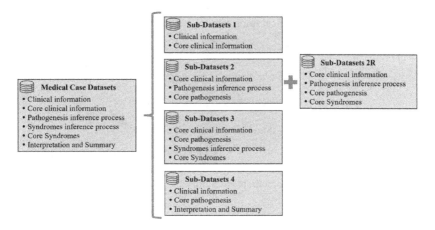

Fig. 2. The medical case dataset is split into four sub-task datasets and one iterative dataset (2R).

4.3   Iterative Retrieval Augmentation Generation Process

Retrieving professional field knowledge and medical case data related to the current subtask can greatly enhance the text quality and syndrome differentiation accuracy generated by pre-trained language models. For example, in the core clinical information extraction subtask, the model can learn which entities are more valuable from the retrieved historical entity extraction cases, thereby improving the quality of the extracted core clinical information. However, there is a problem in this process: We have retrieved and enhanced the quality of the large model's answers for the four subtasks separately, but the interdependence between each task is ignored.

Syndromes can be inferred from pathogenesis and core clinical information, and pathogenesis can also be inferred inversely from syndromes. The relationship between pathogenesis and syndromes is complex. Pathogenesis is the basis of syndromes, and syndromes are the external manifestations of pathogenesis. Changes in pathogenesis will lead to changes in syndromes. Conversely, changes in syndromes can also reflect changes in pathogenesis. The two influence each other. The same disease may exhibit different syndromes at different stages, and different diseases may exhibit similar syndromes at a certain stage. Therefore, the iterative refinement [21, 22] in the framework is reasonable.

As shown in Fig. 3, the specific iterative refinement process is as follows:

1. First, the model extracts core clinical information E from clinical data according to prompts.
2. Based on the extracted core clinical entities E, reasoning is performed to select several possible pathogenesis S for the current case from the given options.

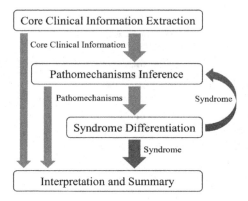

Fig. 3. The collaborative iterative refinement process of sub-tasks.

3. Add the inferred core clinical information E and pathogenesis S to the prompts. The model will infer the possible core syndromes D of the current case based on this information and relevant historical diagnosis data.
4. The framework will refine the pathogenesis S according to the core clinical information E and syndrome D to obtain a more accurate pathogenesis S'. Then use pathogenesis S' to refine the syndrome to obtain D'. Repeat this process continuously until the preset maximum number of iterations is reached.

In order to eliminate the sensitivity of the LLM to the option position when doing multiple-choice questions, we need to randomly rearrange the option positions at each iteration. This helps us obtain better answers.

During the iterative process, the query evolves. After reaching the maximum number of iterations, the loop is exited, achieving more precise retrieval and generating more accurate answers. It is worth noting that the knowledge base retrieved in the first generation process is different from that retrieved later, which is reflected in Fig. 2 (sub-datasets 2 and sub-datasets 2R). This is a cross-link iterative retrieval generation method, which is mainly reflected in the fact that the inference of pathogenesis and syndrome is completed in sequence. During the iterative process, the syndrome is generated based on the pathogenesis, and the query is also evolved according to the syndrome, so as to infer the pathogenesis in reverse.

4.4 Prompt Generation

The importance of prompts for LLMs is self-evident. The performance of the model needs high-quality prompts to guide it so that it can exert its powerful reasoning ability and format the output text. The prompt generation module in the framework mainly considers two prompt technologies: few-shot [28] and chain-of-thought prompting.

Traditional few-shot makes the model learn the same output format as in the examples by giving examples. The examples used in the solution are retrieved from the preprocessed example library. These examples are recalled twice through dense retrieval and sparse retrieval, and then the recalled examples are re-ranked and the three examples that are most in line with the current case are intercepted as prompts. The large model will not only learn the correct output format from these examples but also learn the problem-answer correspondence relationship existing in them. It will be easier to obtain the correct answer.

The chain-of-thought prompting method can give full play to the model's logical reasoning ability and thereby improve its syndrome differentiation ability. The chain-of-thought prompting is specifically carried out through the following three steps:

1. Perform syndrome inference based on historical cases, the patient's core clinical information, and core pathogenesis. Each syndrome must be considered from the three aspects of the patient's symptom manifestations, pulse, and tongue, and cannot be judged one-sidedly;
2. Screen out one or two core syndromes that are most likely to be correct according to syndrome inference;
3. Select the corresponding syndrome answer from the syndrome options according to core syndromes. Separating reasoning and multiple-choice questions helps improve framework performance.

5 Experiments

5.1 Datasets

The dataset is divided into two parts: medical case data and professional knowledge. The medical case data mainly comes from 200 training data provided by the assessment organizer. Professional knowledge mainly comes from the TCM-SD syndrome differentiation dataset [8] in the field of TCM and some classic TCM books. After preprocessing, all these data are used as the knowledge base for retrieval enhancement.

5.2 Evaluation Metrics

The evaluation task examines the performance of the framework from four aspects: core clinical information extraction, pathomechanisms inference, syndrome differentiation, and interpretation and summary. The four subtasks adopt different evaluation indicators due to the nature of the tasks, and finally, the total score is obtained by weighting.

In the core clinical information extraction subtask, the model will extract m clinically relevant entities $E = \{e_1, e_2, ..., e_m\}$, and there is a standard answer $A = \{e'_1, e'_2, ..., e'_n\}$. Then the evaluation index of subtask 1 is:

$$P_1 = \frac{\sum_{i=0}^{m} F(e_i, A)}{n} \tag{1}$$

$$F(e_i, A) = \begin{cases} 0, & if\ e_i \in A \\ 1, & if\ e_i \notin A \end{cases} \tag{2}$$

In the second and third subtasks, the model needs to select k' options from the given k options that match the patient's clinical data. Therefore, the evaluation indicators for these two tasks are:

$$P_2 = P_3 = \frac{n_k}{k + n_k'} \tag{3}$$

n_k is the number of correct options selected by the model, and n_k' is the number of incorrect options selected by the model.

In the subtask of interpreting and summarizing the syndrome differentiation process, the Rouge-L index [29] is used to measure the degree of matching between the summary text and the answer text. This index is widely used to evaluate the quality of text generated by large models. Its calculation method is:

$$R_{LCS} = \frac{LCS(C, S)}{len(S)} \tag{4}$$

$$P_{LCS} = \frac{LCS(C, S)}{len(C)} \tag{5}$$

$$P_4 = \text{Rouge - L} = \frac{(1 + \beta^2)R_{LCS}P_{LCS}}{R_{LCS} + \beta^2 P_{LCS}} \tag{6}$$

The parameter $\beta = 1$. LCS is the longest common subsequence between the interpretation and summary text C given by the model and the answer S.

The final evaluation index is obtained by weighting each subtask and its calculation formula is as follows.

$$P = 20\% \times P_1 + 30\% \times P_2 + 40\% \times P_3 + 10\% \times P_4 \tag{7}$$

5.3   Main Results

The experiment used two general large language models: glm-4-plus and qwen-plus. As can be seen from Table 1, glm-4-plus performs better in the evaluation task. Retrieve 5 related knowledge blocks each time, and after re-ranking them, select 2 of them as examples in the prompts. The number of iterations is set to 7 rounds. This is a trade-off solution that can take into account both time and results.

The technical methods in the framework include Retrieval Augmented Generation(RAG), Chain-of-Thought prompting(CoT), and Reranking technology(rerank). Table 2 shows the evaluation results in round A. All technical methods significantly improve the evaluation score. Taking the most common RAG as the baseline, continuously adding new technologies to improve it, and finally replacing it with Iterative Retrieval Augmented Generation(Iter-RAG).

Table 1. Result of the two rounds

Phase	Large language Model	Score
Round A	glm-4-plus	**30.3406**
	qwen-plus	29.0617
Round B	glm-4-plus	**32.0534**
	qwen-plus	30.5127

Table 2. Best scores of different technical methods in round A. All the other lines calculate Improvement by comparing with the first line.

Technical Method	Score	Improvement
RAG	22.2120	0.0%
RAG + CoT	24.8959	12.08%
RAG + CoT + Rerank	28.5824	28.68%
Iter-RAG + CoT + Rerank	30.3406	36.60%

6   Conclusion

In this paper, we propose a TCM syndrome differentiation framework based on iterative retrieval enhancement technology. This scheme enhances the accuracy of question answering of general LLMs in the professional field of TCM by retrieving medical case data and professional knowledge and reasonably uses the dialectical relationship between pathogenesis and syndromes for their collaborative refinement. In the iteration, it simultaneously improves the accuracy of pathogenesis reasoning and syndrome reasoning. This method shows good performance on a small sample knowledge base. In the TCM syndrome differentiation thinking evaluation task of CHIP2024, the final score reaches 32.0534, ranking fifth among all participating teams, proving the effectiveness of the methodology.

References

1. Zong, H., et al.: Advancing Chinese biomedical text mining with community challenges. J. Biomed. Inf. **157**, 104716 (2024). https://doi.org/10.1016/j.jbi.2024.104716
2. Yang, S., et al.: Zhongjing: enhancing the Chinese medical capabilities of large language model through expert feedback and real-world multi-turn dialogue. In: AAAI Conference on Artificial Intelligence (2023). https://api.semanticscholar.org/CorpusID:260681932
3. Liu, J., Wang, Z., Ye, Q., Chong, D., Zhou, P., Hua, Y.: Qilin-med-vl: towards Chinese large vision-language model for general healthcare. ArXiv arxiv:2310.17956 (2023). https://api.semanticscholar.org/CorpusID:264555208
4. Jin, Y., Chandra, M., Verma, G., Hu, Y., Choudhury, M.D., Kumar, S.: Better to ask in English: cross-lingual evaluation of large language models for healthcare

queries. In: Proceedings of the ACM on Web Conference 2024 (2023). https://api.semanticscholar.org/CorpusID:264405758

5. Qureshi, R.,et al.: Ai in drug discovery and its clinical relevance. Heliyon **9** (2023). https://api.semanticscholar.org/CorpusID:259283533

6. You, Y., et al.: Artificial intelligence in cancer target identification and drug discovery. Signal Transd. Target. Therapy **7** (2022). https://api.semanticscholar.org/CorpusID:248574354

7. Zheng, Y., et al.: Large language models in drug discovery and development: from disease mechanisms to clinical trials. ArXiv arxiv:2409.04481 (2024). https://api.semanticscholar.org/CorpusID:272524743

8. Mucheng, R., Heyan, H., Yuxiang, Z., Qianwen, C., Yuan, B., Yang, G.: TCM-SD: a benchmark for probing syndrome differentiation via natural language processing. In: Sun, M., et al. (eds.) Proceedings of the 21st Chinese National Conference on Computational Linguistics, pp. 908–920. Chinese Information Processing Society of China, Nanchang (2022). https://aclanthology.org/2022.ccl-1.80

9. Zhang, D., Gan, Z., Huang, Z.: Study on classification model of traditional Chinese medicine syndrome types of stroke patients in convalescent stage based on support vector machine. In: 2019 10th International Conference on Information Technology in Medicine and Education (ITME), pp. 205–209. IEEE (2019)

10. Yue, W., et al.: Tcmbench: a comprehensive benchmark for evaluating large language models in traditional chinese medicine. CoRR arxiv:2406.01126 (2024). https://doi.org/10.48550/ARXIV.2406.01126

11. Zhang, H., Wang, X., Meng, Z., Jia, Y., Xu, D.: Qibo: a large language model for traditional Chinese medicine. ArXiv arxiv:2403.16056 (2024). https://api.semanticscholar.org/CorpusID:268681426

12. Zhang, H., Ni, W., Li, J., Zhang, J., et al.: Artificial intelligence-based traditional Chinese medicine assistive diagnostic system: validation study. JMIR Med. Inf. **8**(6), e17608 (2020)

13. Brown, T.B., et al.: Language models are few-shot learners (2020)

14. Raffel, C., et al.: Exploring the limits of transfer learning with a unified text-to-text transformer. J. Mach. Learn. Res. **21**(1) (2020)

15. Touvron, H., et al.: Llama: open and efficient foundation language models. ArXiv arxiv:2302.13971 (2023). https://api.semanticscholar.org/CorpusID:257219404

16. Zhang, X., Tian, C., Yang, X., Chen, L., Li, Z., Petzold, L.R.: Alpacare: instruction-tuned large language models for medical application. ArXiv arxiv:2310.14558 (2023). https://api.semanticscholar.org/CorpusID:264426685

17. Zhu, W., Wang, X., Zheng, H., Chen, M., Tang, B.: Promptcblue: a Chinese prompt tuning benchmark for the medical domain. ArXiv arxiv:2310.14151 (2023). https://api.semanticscholar.org/CorpusID:264426196

18. Wang, X., et al.: Searching for best practices in retrieval-augmented generation. In: Al-Onaizan, Y., Bansal, M., Chen, Y.N. (eds.) Proceedings of the 2024 Conference on Empirical Methods in Natural Language Processing, pp. 17716–17736. Association for Computational Linguistics, Miami (2024). https://aclanthology.org/2024.emnlp-main.981

19. Gao, L., Ma, X., Lin, J., Callan, J.: Precise zero-shot dense retrieval without relevance labels. In: Rogers, A., Boyd-Graber, J., Okazaki, N. (eds.) Proceedings of the 61st Annual Meeting of the Association for Computational Linguistics, vol. 1: Long Papers, pp. 1762–1777. Association for Computational Linguistics, Toronto (2023). https://doi.org/10.18653/v1/2023.acl-long.99. https://aclanthology.org/2023.acl-long.99

20. Chen, T., et al.: Dense X retrieval: what retrieval granularity should we use? In: Al-Onaizan, Y., Bansal, M., Chen, Y.N. (eds.) Proceedings of the 2024 Conference on Empirical Methods in Natural Language Processing, pp. 15159–15177. Association for Computational Linguistics, Miami (2024). https://aclanthology.org/2024.emnlp-main.845

21. Trivedi, H., Balasubramanian, N., Khot, T., Sabharwal, A.: Interleaving retrieval with chain-of-thought reasoning for knowledge-intensive multi-step questions. ArXiv arxiv:2212.10509 (2022). https://api.semanticscholar.org/CorpusID: 254877499

22. Sarthi, P., Abdullah, S., Tuli, A., Khanna, S., Goldie, A., Manning, C.D.: Raptor: recursive abstractive processing for tree-organized retrieval. ArXiv arxiv:2401.18059 (2024). https://api.semanticscholar.org/CorpusID:267334785

23. Zheng, H.S., et al.: Take a step back: evoking reasoning via abstraction in large language models. ArXiv arxiv:2310.06117 (2023). https://api.semanticscholar.org/CorpusID:263830368

24. Wei, J., et al.: Chain-of-thought prompting elicits reasoning in large language models. In: Koyejo, S., Mohamed, S., Agarwal, A., Belgrave, D., Cho, K., Oh, A. (eds.) Advances in Neural Information Processing Systems, vol. 35, pp. 24824–24837. Curran Associates, Inc. (2022). https://proceedings.neurips.cc/paper_files/paper/2022/file/9d5609613524ecf4f15af0f7b31abca4-Paper-Conference.pdf

25. Sun, J., et al.: Enhancing chain-of-thoughts prompting with iterative bootstrapping in large language models. In: Duh, K., Gomez, H., Bethard, S. (eds.) Findings of the Association for Computational Linguistics: NAACL 2024, pp. 4074–4101. Association for Computational Linguistics, Mexico City (2024). https://doi.org/10.18653/v1/2024.findings-naacl.257. https://aclanthology.org/2024.findings-naacl.257

26. Kojima, T., Gu, S.S., Reid, M., Matsuo, Y., Iwasawa, Y.: Large language models are zero-shot reasoners. In: Koyejo, S., Mohamed, S., Agarwal, A., Belgrave, D., Cho, K., Oh, A. (eds.) Advances in Neural Information Processing Systems, vol. 35, pp. 22199–22213. Curran Associates, Inc. (2022). https://proceedings.neurips.cc/paper_files/paper/2022/file/8bb0d291acd4acf06ef112099c16f326-Paper-Conference.pdf

27. Williams, A.: Comparison of generative ai performance on undergraduate and postgraduate written assessments in the biomedical sciences. Int. J. Educ. Technol. High. Educ. 21(1), 52 (2024)

28. Sanh, V., et al.: Multitask prompted training enables zero-shot task generalization. ArXiv arxiv:2110.08207 (2021). https://api.semanticscholar.org/CorpusID: 239009562

29. Lin, C.Y.: ROUGE: a package for automatic evaluation of summaries. In: Text Summarization Branches Out, pp. 74–81. Association for Computational Linguistics, Barcelona (2004). https://aclanthology.org/W04-1013

Lymphoma Information Extraction and Automatic Coding

Benchmark for Lymphoma Information Extraction and Automated Coding

Hui Zong[1], Liang Tao[2]($\boxtimes$), Zuofeng Li[3], Chunxiao Wu[4], Yuxian Liu[5], and Xiaoyan Zhang[3]

[1] West China Hospital, Sichuan University, Chengdu, Sichuan, China
[2] Faculty of Business Information, Shanghai Business School, Shanghai, China
tao.liang@msn.com
[3] School of Life Sciences and Technology, Tongji University, Shanghai, China
[4] Shanghai Municipal Center for Disease Control and Prevention, Shanghai, China
[5] Tongji University Library, Tongji University, Shanghai, China

Abstract. We present a specialized dataset for automated lymphoma coding, comprising 162 case reports sourced from Chinese Medical Case Repository website. Each report is coded according to the ICD-O-3 and ICD-10 classification systems for both Hodgkin lymphoma and non-Hodgkin lymphoma cases. The dataset is strategically divided into three equal parts: a training set of 54 reports, and two test sets (A and B) containing 54 case reports each, providing a foundation for developing and evaluating large language models in oncology coding. Our resource is designed to facilitate advancements in automated tumor coding systems, with the potential to significantly enhance the efficiency and accuracy of lymphoma classification in clinical settings. The dataset, along with comprehensive evaluation metrics, is accessible at http://cips-chip.org.cn/2024/eval2. It serves as a valuable tool for researchers and practitioners in medical informatics and oncology, particularly those focusing on Chinese language medical texts and international classification guidelines.

Keywords: Clinical Coding · ICD-O · ICD · Lymphoma

1 Introduction

Lymphoma is a prevalent group of malignant neoplasms originating in the lymphatic system. It is broadly categorized into two main types: Hodgkin lymphoma (HL) and non-Hodgkin lymphoma (NHL). Hodgkin lymphoma typically has a favorable prognosis and is often curable with appropriate treatment. In contrast, the prognosis for non-Hodgkin lymphoma varies significantly depending on the specific subtype. The diverse nature of NHL subtypes leads to a wide range of clinical outcomes, with some forms being highly aggressive while others follow a more indolent course. This heterogeneity in NHL underscores the importance of

© The Author(s), under exclusive license to Springer Nature Singapore Pte Ltd. 2025
Y. Zhang et al. (Eds.): CHIP 2024, CCIS 2458, pp. 67–74, 2025.
https://doi.org/10.1007/978-981-96-4298-4_6

accurate diagnosis and subtyping for determining the most effective treatment approach and predicting patient outcomes.

According to estimates by the International Agency for Research on Cancer of the World Health Organization [1, 2], in 2022, there were approximately 553,000 new cases of NHL globally, ranking 10th in cancer incidence. The mortality rate was 7.0 per 100,000, with an age-standardized incidence rate of 5.6 per 100,000. In the same year, about 251,000 people died from NHL, ranking 11th in cancer-related deaths. The mortality rate was 3.2 per 100,000, with an age-standardized mortality rate of 2.4 per 100,000.

In 2022, there were 85,000 new cases of lymphoma in China [3], ranking 13th in cancer incidence. The incidence rate was 6.03 per 100,000, with an age-standardized incidence rate of 3.77 per 100,000. In the same year, 41,600 people died from lymphoma in China, ranking 11th in cancer-related deaths. The mortality rate was 2.95 per 100,000, with an age-standardized mortality rate of 1.64 per 100,000.

Clinical diagnosis coding is the process of converting clinical diagnostic information, such as case reports, into a standardized and unified coding system. This process facilitates the recording, statistical analysis, and examination of medical data, as well as communication between clinical information recorded in different languages. For example, the currently most widely used ICD-10 (International Statistical Classification of Diseases and Related Health Problems, 10th Revision) coding system serves as a standardized tool for various normalized medical and epidemiological statistics, including hospital medical records, death registrations, and various disease surveillance activities.

The purpose of clinical diagnosis coding is multifaceted. It enables efficient recording of medical data, facilitates statistical analysis of health information, allows for comprehensive analysis of medical data, and promotes communication and comparison of clinical information across different languages and healthcare systems. By using a standardized coding system like ICD-10, healthcare professionals and researchers can achieve several important objectives. They can maintain consistency in medical record-keeping and conduct accurate epidemiological studies. Furthermore, this standardization enables them to monitor disease trends and patterns effectively. It also allows for the comparison of health data across different regions and countries, ultimately leading to improvements in the overall quality of healthcare delivery and public health management.

This standardization plays a crucial role in advancing medical research, enhancing patient care, and informing health policy decisions on both national and international levels. It provides a common language for healthcare providers, researchers, and policymakers, allowing for more effective collaboration and decision-making in the field of public health. By ensuring that medical information is recorded and analyzed in a consistent manner across different healthcare systems and geographical areas, this standardization contributes significantly to the global effort to improve health outcomes and address health challenges more efficiently.

2   Lymphoma Dataset

2.1   Description

Around the year 2000, China's hospital medical records, cause of death registration, and various disease surveillance systems generally transitioned from ICD-9 to ICD-10 for disease coding. ICD-10 remains the standard in China today. Similarly, ICD-O (International Classification of Diseases for Oncology) is primarily used for cancer registration and pathological coding. It was first established in 1976. In 1998, Shanghai began using ICD-O-2. In 2002, Shanghai became the first region in mainland China to fully implement ICD-O-2 coding. In 2008, Shanghai upgraded to ICD-O-3. Apart from hospitals in the Shanghai region, a limited number of hospitals in other regions of China have also adopted ICD-O-3 specifically for coding cancer-related diseases.

The Shanghai Municipal Center for Disease Control and Prevention (briefly as Shanghai CDC) has made significant contributions to tumor coding based on their experience using ICD-10 and ICD-O-3 in conjunction. They have systematically explored the inherent patterns and summarized coding methods, facilitating the publication of a reference book titled *Tumor Nomenclature and Coding*. This comprehensive guide has gained widespread recognition and appreciation from peers across China, establishing Shanghai as a leader in the field of tumor coding.

In a demonstration of their commitment to staying at the forefront of international standards, the Shanghai CDC rapidly responded to the release of ICD-O-3.2 in 2018. They swiftly completed the Chinese translation and necessary updates of this new version in a very short timeframe. Subsequently, in 2020, the translated and updated version of ICD-O-3.2 was officially implemented throughout Shanghai, further solidifying the city's position as a pioneer in adopting and adapting advanced tumor coding systems.

Clearly, the application of ICD-O-3 coding significantly enhances the precision of tumor classification and downstream statistical analysis. This advanced coding system enables researchers and clinicians to conduct studies on specific pathological types of tumors and perform statistical analyses based on pathological classifications, which was previously challenging or impossible. For instance, ICD-O-3 coding allows for detailed analysis of different pathological types of lung cancer and their impact on survival rates. This level of granularity provides valuable insights into the nature of lung cancer and can inform more targeted treatment approaches. In addition, ICD-O-3 facilitates research on less common tumor types, such as gastrointestinal stromal tumors (GISTs). By providing a standardized and detailed coding system for these specific tumor types, ICD-O-3 supports in-depth studies that can advance our understanding of these particular cancers and potentially lead to improved treatment strategies.

2.2   Lymphoma Automated Coding

In this year's evaluation of China Health Information Processing Conference (CHIP), our primary task is to explore the potential of large language models for automatic information extraction and tumor coding related to lymphoma. Unlike solid tumor coding, which only records the site, the ICD-10 (latest 2019 version) introduced pathological types into its coding system for precise classification of lymphomas, leukemias, and other lymphohematopoietic system tumors. This addition has increased the complexity of the coding system, resulting in the establishment of 7 categories and 48 distinct codes for lymphohematopoietic system tumors. In parallel, the ICD-O-3 (International Classification of Diseases for Oncology, 3rd Edition, latest 2nd revision), which is specifically designed for cancer registration, has set up 66 corresponding pathological morphology codes for lymphohematopoietic system tumors.

Consequently, this requires higher medical expertise from coding personnel, making the task more challenging and time-consuming. Exploring large language models can greatly improve the speed of tumor coding while enhancing the accuracy of automatic tumor coding.

This task holds significant importance for several reasons. First, it addresses the complexity of lymphoma coding in modern classification systems. Furthermore, it acknowledges the higher level of medical knowledge required for accurate coding, highlighting the specialized expertise needed in this field. The task also takes into account the time-consuming nature of manual coding processes, which can be a bottleneck in efficient healthcare data management. Importantly, this task proposes the use of large language models as a potential solution to improve both speed and accuracy in tumor coding. This innovative approach aims to contribute to more efficient and precise cancer registration and statistics.

By leveraging the capabilities of large language models, this research could potentially revolutionize the field of medical coding, particularly for complex cases like lymphomas. The implications of this work are far-reaching, as it could lead to more timely and accurate cancer statistics. These improved statistics are invaluable for oncological research, healthcare planning, and policy-making. Ultimately, this advancement in medical coding technology could contribute to better patient care, more effective resource allocation in healthcare systems, and more informed decision-making in public health policies related to cancer management and prevention.

While there have been various research papers on ICD-10 and ICD-O-3 coding [4], our focus is specifically on the ICD-O-3 lymphoma coding task. The ICD-O has been applied in cancer registration and tumor pathology statistics for over 30 years globally, with more than a decade of foundation in China. Importantly, ICD-O-3 can be perfectly converted to ICD-10, but the reverse could be not possible. Based on the current practical application scenario of the Shanghai CDC, cancer registration work still adheres to the method of using both ICD-10 and ICD-O-3 coding systems in conjunction, as shown in Table 1. It's worth noting that while the ICD-10 has been updated to the 2019 version, and despite WHO's recommendation to adopt ICD-11, the actual application of ICD-11 remains limited in China.

Table 1. Coding Structure

I: ICD-10 Coding		
C _	_	._
I ①	②	.③
C 8	3	.3

II: ICD-O-3 Topography Coding		
C _	_	._
II ①	②	.③
C 4	2	. 1

III: ICD-O-3 Morphology, Behavior and Differentiation Coding					
M- _	_	_	_	/ _	_
III ①	②	③	④	/⑤	⑥
M-9	6	8	0	/3	6

2.3 Data Collection and Statistics

A comprehensive data collection process was undertaken to gather information on lymphoma from a Chinese Medical Case Repository website. The research began by conducting a search using the keyword "淋巴瘤" (lymphoma) on the website https://cmcr.yiigle.com/index. This initial search yielded a substantial result set of 2,880 documents, providing a rich source of case reports for the study.

Then a custom web crawler was designed to navigate the search results and extract the XML web pages, including three key pieces of information: the URL, the title, and the full text content. This ensured that the most relevant and useful information was captured for downstream analysis of automated coding.

From the total collection of extracted documents, 200 were randomly selected to serve as the annotation set. The annotation process was conducted using the *Tumor Nomenclature and Coding* book by the Shanghai CDC. This book has been designed with a primary focus on facilitating the coding process for registrars, whose distinctive feature lies in the integration of topography codes from both ICD-10 and ICD-O-3, creating a unified reference system. Further, the three-way correspondence between ICD-10 and ICD-O-3 topography codes, along with pathological codes is highlighted especially for coding lymphohematopoietic systems. This strategic alignment serves a dual purpose: it streamlines the code lookup process for registrars while simultaneously reducing the likelihood of coding errors. This book clearly serves as a standardized guide for tumor coding in the region, ensuring consistency and accuracy in the annotation process.

The annotation task was carried out by a highly experienced expert with over two decades of experience in tumor coding and registration. Notably, this expert was also the lead author of the *Tumor Nomenclature and Coding* book, bringing expertise to the annotation process. This level of experience and familiarity with the coding system significantly enhances the reliability and validity of the annotations. The annotation process was thorough and time-intensive, spanning over one month. This extended period allowed for careful consideration of each document, ensuring high-quality annotations of lymphoma coding.

Following the annotation, a screening process was implemented to refine the dataset. Two primary exclusion criteria were applied: 1) case reports unrelated to lymphoma were removed to maintain the focus of the dataset. 2) documents describing two or more patients were excluded to ensure each data point corresponded to a single, distinct case. This screening process resulted in a final dataset of 162 documents, each representing a unique and relevant lymphoma case.

In what follows, the curated dataset was strategically divided into three distinct subsets to facilitate the development and evaluation of the model. The training set comprises 54 case reports, serving as the primary corpus for model training and learning. This subset is crucial for the model to learn patterns and features associated with lymphoma coding. For comprehensive model evaluation, two separate test sets were created: Test Set A and Test Set B. Each of these test sets contains 54 case reports, mirroring the size of the training set. This balanced distribution ensures a robust evaluation process. Test Set A is typically used for initial model assessment and potential fine-tuning, while Test Set B serves as a final evaluation benchmark, often reserved for assessing the model's generalization capabilities on unseen data. It's important to note that across these three subsets, the entire curated dataset encompasses approximately 30 unique morphology codes, representing about half of the total morphology codes used in lymphoma coding.

This tripartite division of the dataset adheres to best practices in machine learning, allowing for effective model training, validation, and unbiased performance assessment. The equal size of each subset (54 case reports) provides a balanced approach to model development and evaluation. This approach to annotation and dataset curation demonstrates a commitment to creating a high-quality, focused dataset. The combination of expert annotation, standardized coding guidelines, and careful screening enhances the dataset's potential utility for subsequent statistical analysis and machine learning applications in the field of lymphoma research and coding.

2.4   Limitations

The dataset used in this study, while valuable, presents several limitations that warrant consideration. Foremost is the constraint of sample size. With only 162 case reports, the dataset is relatively small, which may potentially impact the model's ability to generalize effectively to a broader range of cases. This limited sample size could lead to challenges in capturing the full spectrum of variability present in lymphoma cases.

Another limitation lies in the potential lack of diversity in lymphoma subtypes represented within the dataset. It is possible that not all subtypes of lymphoma are adequately represented, with some subtypes potentially having very few examples. This imbalance in subtype representation could lead to biases in the model's performance across different lymphoma categories.

The dataset's homogeneity in terms of its source is another point of consideration. As the case reports were collected from a single source, they may not fully represent the true diversity of lymphoma cases across the entire country. This lack of geographical and institutional diversity in the data source could limit the model's applicability to cases from different regions or healthcare settings.

Lastly, the human element in the annotation process introduces the possibility of subjective bias. Despite the high expertise of the annotator, the inherent subjectivity in interpretation and coding decisions cannot be entirely eliminated. This potential for human bias in the annotation process could lead to inconsistencies or systematic errors in the coded data, which in turn might influence the model's learning and subsequent coding performance.

3   Discussion and Future Work

This dataset holds significant potential for advancing the field of automated tumor coding systems. By facilitating the development and evaluation of large language models in oncology coding, it serves as a crucial stepping stone towards more sophisticated automated coding systems. This progression is expected to have a transformative impact on the efficiency and accuracy of tumor registration processes.

The practical implications of this research extend directly to clinical settings. By paving the way for automated coding procedures, this dataset contributes to enhancing the productivity and precision of coding professionals. This automation not only streamlines workflow but also potentially reduces human error, leading to more reliable and consistent coding outcomes in oncology.

The experimental results derived from this dataset provide valuable insights for future improvements. These findings can guide refinements in data collection methodologies and model architectures, ultimately enhancing the accuracy and applicability of coding systems. Such iterative improvements are essential for developing robust, real-world solutions that can adapt to the complexities and nuances of clinical oncology coding.

Looking ahead, this research task holds profound implications for the broader application of large language models in clinical information extraction and coding. It serves as a proof of concept for the potential of large language models in efficiently handling tumor clinical information extraction and automated coding. The insights gained from this study could inform future developments in large language models applications within healthcare, particularly in areas requiring high-level interpretation of medical narratives.

This work represents a step towards integrating advanced language foundation models into routine clinical practice, potentially revolutionizing how medical information is organized, coded, and understood in oncology and beyond. As such, it not only addresses current challenges in automated coding assistance but also sets the stage for broader innovations in real-time diagnostic suggestions and tailored treatment protocols.

Acknowledgments. This work was supported by the National Social Science Fund of China (grant number 72274139).

References

1. Global Cancer Observatory: Cancer Today (2024). https://gco.iarc.fr/today/en/dataviz/tables?mode=population&group_populations=0&cancers=34. Accessed 15 Nov 2024
2. Bray, F., et al.: Global cancer statistics 2022: GLOBOCAN estimates of incidence and mortality worldwide for 36 cancers in 185 countries. CA Cancer J. Clin. **74**(3), 229–263 (2024). https://doi.org/10.3322/caac.21834
3. Han, B., et al.: Cancer incidence and mortality in China, 2022. J. Natl. Cancer Center **4**(1), 47–53 (2024). https://doi.org/10.1016/j.jncc.2024.01.006
4. Zong, H., et al.: Advancing Chinese biomedical text mining with community challenges. J. Biomed. Inform. **157**, 104716 (2024). https://doi.org/10.1016/j.jbi.2024.104716. tex.ids= zong_advancing_2024-1

Overview of the Lymphoma Information Extraction and Automatic Coding Evaluation Task in CHIP 2024

Hui Zong[1], Liang Tao[2(✉)], Zuofeng Li[3], Chunxiao Wu[4], Yuxian Liu[5], and Xiaoyan Zhang[3]

[1] West China Hospital, Sichuan University, Chengdu 610041, Sichuan, China
[2] Faculty of Business Information, Shanghai Business School, Shanghai 201400, China
tao.liang@msn.com
[3] School of Life Sciences and Technology, Tongji University, Shanghai 200092, China
[4] Shanghai Municipal Center for Disease Control and Prevention, Shanghai 200336, China
[5] Tongji University Library, Tongji University, Shanghai 200092, China

Abstract. Lymphoma diagnostic coding is vital for streamlining clinical documentation and supporting tumor registries. This paper introduces the "Lymphoma Information Extraction and Automatic Coding Task," organized at CHIP 2024, to evaluate the performance of large language models (LLMs) in generating tumor registry codes based on ICD-10 and ICD-O-3 standards. The dataset, comprising 162 clinical case reports, was divided into training set, test set A and test set B. The task assessed accuracy across three coding types, with leaderboard evaluations highlighting innovative approaches. Accuracy is used as evaluation metric. Eighteen participating teams submitted their solutions, with the top-ranked team achieving a score of 0.9296. The top-ranked teams employed diverse methodologies, including LLMs fine-tuning, structured pipelines, Chain of Thought reasoning, and retrieval-augmented generation frameworks, achieving impressive results. This paper provides insights into the dataset, evaluation metrics, and top-performing solutions, offering a foundation for advancing automated medical coding with LLMs.

Keywords: Large language model · Retrieval-augmented Generation · Lymphoma · Information extraction · ICD · CHIP

1 Introduction

Lymphoma is a malignant tumor originating from the abnormal proliferation of lymphocytes or lymphatic tissues within the lymphatic system [1]. It is primarily categorized into two major types: Hodgkin lymphoma and non-Hodgkin lymphoma, both of which exhibit a high incidence globally [2, 3]. Clinical diagnostic coding is a critical process that translates diagnostic information into standardized codes, facilitating the recording, communication, and analysis of medical data [4]. By providing a unified framework, this process ensures the accuracy, consistency, and comparability of healthcare information.

© The Author(s), under exclusive license to Springer Nature Singapore Pte Ltd. 2025
Y. Zhang et al. (Eds.): CHIP 2024, CCIS 2458, pp. 75–84, 2025.
https://doi.org/10.1007/978-981-96-4298-4_7

In the clinical diagnosis of lymphoma, physicians must integrate multiple sources of information, including patient history, physical examination, laboratory tests, imaging studies, and, most importantly, pathological findings, to produce a comprehensive evaluation and encode the diagnosis accordingly. However, the complexity and heterogeneity of lymphoma, characterized by numerous subtypes with distinct clinical features and diagnostic criteria, make this coding process challenging.

In recent years, large language models (LLMs) have demonstrated significant potential in medical applications [5], particularly in the domain of clinical diagnostic coding for lymphoma. By leveraging extensive medical literature, case reports, and clinical guidelines, these models can acquire profound medical knowledge. They are capable of autonomously analyzing and interpreting complex clinical information, offering precise coding recommendations. LLMs can effectively emulate the reasoning process of human coders, providing personalized and intelligent coding solutions that support more accurate decision-making.

To explore the performance of LLMs in comprehensive tumor registry coding for lymphoma, we introduced the Lymphoma Information Extraction and Automatic Coding Task at the China Health Information Processing Conference (CHIP). The CHIP [6], organized by the Special Interest Committee on Medical Health and Bioinformation Processing under the Chinese Information Processing Society of China, is an annual conference and one of the most prominent academic events in the field of health information processing in China. The CHIP conference focuses on interdisciplinary areas such as medical informatics, health informatics, and bioinformatics, bringing together researchers and professionals from academia, industry, and government worldwide to share cutting-edge research, innovative ideas, and successful practices. This task focuses on assessing the accuracy and efficiency of tumor coding, aiming to evaluate the disparities between LLM-generated and human-coded results, analyze their respective strengths and limitations, and further promote the integration of LLMs into clinical practice. This paper provides an in-depth overview of the task. First, we present the task's background and review relevant research. Next, we describe the overall design, characteristics of the dataset, and evaluation metrics. Finally, we summarize the task implementation, and offer detailed insights into the algorithms and optimization strategies employed by the top five participating teams.

2 Related Works

The automatic assignment of diagnostic codes, such as ICD-10 or ICD-O, is a crucial task in healthcare informatics, streamlining the process of clinical documentation and enabling efficient medical data management. Over the years, research has progressed from traditional rule-based systems to more sophisticated methods, including machine learning, neural networks, and, most recently, pre-trained and large language models.

Traditional rule-based systems relied on predefined sets of rules and semantic matching to assign codes based on structured and unstructured clinical data. These systems often incorporated keyword matching, regular expressions, and ontological reasoning to extract and map relevant information [7]. While effective in controlled environments, they struggled with ambiguous, incomplete, or nuanced language in clinical notes, limiting their scalability and robustness. Early work such as the construction of rule-based ICD coding systems highlighted the foundational importance of this approach [8, 9].

The advent of machine learning introduced significant improvements in automated coding by leveraging statistical patterns within large datasets. Supervised learning models were widely adopted, particularly for tasks like ICD-10 and ICD-9 coding. Systems based on algorithms such as support vector machines and logistic regression demonstrated increased flexibility compared to rule-based methods. For example, semi-automatic systems and supervised neural networks enhanced coding accuracy by learning from labeled data [10, 11]. Despite these advancements, traditional ML models required extensive feature engineering, which limited their adaptability to complex and diverse datasets.

Deep learning methods represented a paradigm shift, enabling the automatic extraction of hierarchical features from unstructured clinical text [12]. Architectures such as BiRNN, CNNs, and attention mechanisms became popular for medical coding tasks, significantly outperforming earlier methods in terms of accuracy and scalability [12–15]. Attention-based neural architectures further improved the interpretability of automated coding models by focusing on relevant parts of the input text. Notably, systems employing multilayer attention BiRNN and deep transfer learning demonstrated exceptional performance in the automatic assignment of ICD codes by leveraging context.

Recent developments in LLMs, such as GPT-based architectures, have shown great promise in automating disease coding tasks [16]. With their immense scale and ability to handle complex natural language queries, LLMs have significantly advanced the state of the art in clinical NLP. Studies have demonstrated the application of LLMs for tasks such as retina ICD coding and inpatient diagnosis coding, highlighting their versatility and potential for domain adaptation [17]. Despite these advances, benchmarking studies have revealed limitations in their performance, particularly in terms of medical-specific reasoning and code accuracy, emphasizing the need for further refinement [18].

3 Dataset

3.1 Task Definition

The task involves automatic clinical coding for case reports of lymphoma patients. These reports typically include information such as patient demographics, clinical examinations, diagnoses, and treatments. The objective is to assign the corresponding clinical diagnostic codes to each case, based on the Tumor Nomenclature and Coding guidelines, published by the Shanghai Municipal Center for Disease Control and Prevention (1st edition, November 2022, Shanghai Popular Science Press). The tumor coding system integrates both ICD-10 and ICD-O-3 standards and is divided into three distinct parts, as illustrated in Fig. 1.

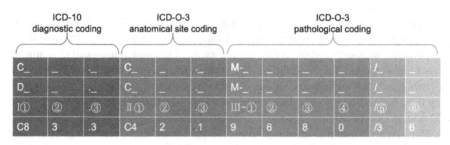

Fig. 1. The structure of coding.

The tumor coding system comprises three main components. The first component is the ICD-10 coding, represented by sections ①–③, which correspond to the ICD-10 diagnostic codes. The second component is the ICD-O-3 anatomical site coding, also represented by sections ①–③, which encode the anatomical location of the tumor based on the ICD-O-3 standard. The third component is the ICD-O-3 pathological coding, which includes multiple sections: sections ①–④ are used for ICD-O-3 morphological coding, section ⑤ is designated for ICD-O-3 behavioral coding, and section ⑥ represents the ICD-O-3 histological grade and differentiation coding. Detailed descriptions of behavioral coding and histological grade coding can be found in Tables 1 and 2, respectively.

Table 1. The description of behavioral coding.

Code	Meaning
/0	Benign
/1	Uncertain whether benign or malignant/borderline; low malignant potential/uncertain malignant potential
/2	In situ tumor/intraepithelial/non-invasive/non-infiltrative
/3	Malignant, primary site
/6	Malignant, metastatic site/malignant, secondary site
/9	Malignant, uncertain whether primary or metastatic site

3.2 Dataset Description

The dataset for this task originates from published clinical case reports in Chinese medical literature. A total of 162 case reports related to lymphoma were curated, and these were split into three subsets. The training set with 54 reports, the test set A with 54 reports, used for model debugging during the competition, and the test set B with 54 reports, reserved for final task evaluation and ranking. A dataset sample is shown in Fig. 2.

Table 2. The description of histological grade coding. Note: Codes 5–8 apply exclusively to lymphoma and leukemia (M-9590~9989).

Code	Meaning
1	Grade I/Well-differentiated/Differentiated, NOS
2	Grade II/Moderately differentiated/Intermediate differentiation
3	Grade III/Poorly differentiated
4	Grade IV/Undifferentiated/Anaplastic
5	T-cell
6	B-cell/Pre-B/B-precursor cell
7	Null lymphocyte/Non-T, Non-B
8	NK (Natural Killer) cell
9	Grade or differentiation unspecified, not stated, or not applicable; cell type unspecified, not stated, or not applicable

```
{
  "id": "s001",
  "text": "'噬血细胞综合征 (hemophagocytic syndrome, HPS) 又称噬血细胞性淋巴组织细胞增多症
      一、一般资料
      患者，女性，60岁，因"头晕乏力1个月余，发热1 d"入院．患者1个月前......
      二、检查．
      2023年3月8日血常规:血红蛋白54 g/L;血小板计数77x10 9/L......
      三、诊断与鉴别诊断
      根据上述结果最终诊断: 1.弥漫大B细胞淋巴瘤IV期 (AnnArbor 4B期IPI 4分......
      四、治疗
      患者初诊考虑为Evans综合征，激素治疗有效，随访中出现血小板及血红蛋白......
      五、治疗结果、随访及转归
      患者经R-CHOP方案4个疗程评估后达到CR，目前化疗......'",
  "date_of_first_diagnosis": "2023年6月15日",
  "gender": "女",
  "location": "骨髓",
  "pathological_classification": "弥漫大B细胞性非霍奇金淋巴瘤累及骨髓IV期，",
  "ICD-10":"C83.3",
  "ICD-O-P":"C42.1",
  "ICD-O-M":"9680/3",
  "ICD-O-H":"6"
}
```

Fig. 2. An example of dataset.

The dataset includes the following components:

text: A comprehensive narrative describing the patient's history, including demographic details, clinical manifestations, examination results, diagnostic process, treatment plan, outcomes, and follow-up.

date_of_first_diagnosis: The date when the patient was first diagnosed with lymphoma.
gender: The patient's gender.
location: The anatomical location of the tumor.

pathological_classification: The pathological staging information.
ICD-10: The ICD-10 code for the diagnosis.
ICD-O-P: The ICD-O-3 anatomical site code.
ICD-O-M: The combined ICD-O-3 morphological and behavioral codes.
ICD-O-H: The ICD-O-3 histological grade and differentiation code.

The input to the model is the case report narrative text, while other components such as date_of_first_diagnosis, gender, location, and pathological_classification are supplementary and aid the coding process. The output includes the predicted codes: ICD-10, ICD-O-M, and ICD-O-H. The model's output must be formatted as a UTF-8 encoded JSON file. While all extracted components should be included in the submission, only the accuracy of the coding predictions for ICD-10, ICD-O-M, and ICD-O-H are considered for the model evaluation and ranking, with weights of 0.3, 0.5, and 0.2, respectively.

3.3 Evaluation Metrics

The evaluation of the task focuses exclusively on the accuracy of the automatic coding predictions. The final ranking score is computed as a weighted sum of accuracies for the three evaluated code types:

ICD-10 Coding Accuracy (Accuracy-ICD-10): The proportion of correct ICD-10 predictions across all samples, weighted at 0.3.
ICD-O-3 Morphological and Behavioral Coding Accuracy (Accuracy-ICD-O-M): The proportion of correct ICD-O-M predictions, weighted at 0.5.
ICD-O-3 Histological Grade and Differentiation Coding Accuracy (Accuracy-ICD-O-H): The proportion of correct ICD-O-H predictions, weighted at 0.2.

The final score is calculated as:

$$Accuracy = 0.3 \times Accuracy_{ICD-10} + 0.5 \times Accuracy_{ICD-O-M} + 0.2 \times Accuracy_{ICD-O-H}$$

Each component's accuracy is determined as follows:

$$Accuracy_{ICD-10} = \frac{Number\ of\ correct\ ICD - 10\ predictions}{Total\ number\ of\ samples}$$

$$Accuracy_{ICD-O-M} = \frac{Number\ of\ correct\ ICD - O - M\ predictions}{Total\ number\ of\ samples}$$

$$Accuracy_{ICD-O-H} = \frac{Number\ of\ correct\ ICD - O - H\ predictions}{Total\ number\ of\ samples}$$

The final ranking score is the mean weighted accuracy across all samples, reflecting the model's overall performance in automated clinical coding.

4 Results

4.1 Overview

This task comprises two distinct phases: the initial round (leaderboard A) and the final round (leaderboard B). Leaderboard A lasted for a month, while leaderboard B spanned five days. The statistical details of the results are presented in Table 3. In leaderboard A, a total of 25 submissions were received from participating teams. The maximum value recorded was 0.8685. For leaderboard B, there were 18 submissions from participating teams, with the highest value being 0.9296. The average score was 0.7284, with a median of 0.7787.

Table 3. Statistical description of all submissions.

Phase	Submissions	Max	Min	Average	Median
leaderboard A	25	0.8685	0.0685	0.6065	0.6555
leaderboard B	18	0.9296	0.0241	0.7284	0.7787

4.2 Top Five Solutions

Table 4 shows the performance of the top five teams in leaderboard B of this task. Here we briefly introduce the methods used by the top five teams.

Table 4. The performance results of top five ranking teams.

Ranking	Score	ICD-10	ICD-O-M	ICD-O-H
1st	0.9296	0.9259	0.9259	0.9444
2nd	0.9222	0.8889	0.9259	0.9630
3th	0.8963	0.9074	0.9074	0.8519
4th	0.8926	0.8704	0.9074	0.8889
5th	0.8704	0.8519	0.8889	0.8519

The first-ranked team proposed an innovative method for automatic ICD coding of lymphoma using LLMs, achieving a comprehensive score of 92.96%. Their approach integrates three main stages: Disease Code Mapping Table Construction, Automatic Prompt Engineering (APE), and the ReAct framework. In the mapping table construction stage, structured and unstructured data are harmonized using LLMs, with a Chinese-English disease name mapping strategy ensuring consistency. Data heterogeneity is addressed by extracting key information from unstructured text and aligning English and Chinese terminology with semantic equivalence. The APE stage automates the generation and optimization of high-quality prompts. Using forward and reverse modes, candidate prompts are generated, filtered iteratively, and expanded with semantically similar samples to maximize performance. Finally, the ReAct framework combines reasoning and action steps to enhance coding accuracy and efficiency. By reasoning through diagnosis, matching diseases, and mapping to standardized codes (ICD-10, ICD-O-3), the method dynamically refines its actions based on real-time feedback, ensuring robust decision-making and adaptability. This comprehensive framework underscores the potential of LLMs in addressing the complexities of clinical coding for heterogeneous diseases like lymphoma.

The second-ranked team proposed a robust approach to automate lymphoma diagnostic coding using a self-developed medical LLM combined with a structured pipeline. Their methodology involved three main steps: lymphoma information extraction, encoding retrieval, and post-processing. For information extraction, they utilized prompt engineering integrated with the Retrieval-Augmented Generation (RAG) approach, specifically employing GraphRAG to process case reports structurally and extract key pathological staging data. To enhance retrieval accuracy, a coarse-to-fine ranking method was applied, leveraging keyword and semantic vector search to match extracted tumor staging data with database records. Post-processing involved a mutual mapping strategy, exploiting the inherent relationships between ICD-10 and ICD-O-M codes to improve coding precision. Additionally, the team implemented a Multi-Vec Retrieval mechanism to capture nuanced text similarities by transforming text into multi-dimensional vector representations, enabling fine-grained semantic matching. This comprehensive pipeline effectively simulated human cognitive processes in coding, demonstrating the potential for LLMs in clinical applications while addressing the challenges posed by the diversity and complexity of lymphoma subtypes.

The third-ranked team proposed a method leveraging Chain of Thought (CoT) reasoning with LLMs to enhance the accuracy and interpretability of automated ICD coding for lymphoma cases. Their approach comprised three main modules: diagnosis extraction, ICD knowledge-based curation, and CoT prompt development. They designed structured prompts to guide LLMs in extracting diagnostic terms and mapping them to corresponding ICD-10 and ICD-O codes. To ensure precision, their prompts included task descriptions, output formats, and examples. The team curated an updated ICD knowledge base to mitigate LLMs' limitations in medical domain expertise and address issues like hallucinations. They further optimized CoT prompts to emulate the step-by-step reasoning of human coders, systematically extracting keywords, matching them to a lymphoma-specific code mapping table, and selecting the most relevant codes. This method demonstrated improved accuracy with model-specific CoT customization, highlighting its potential for scalable and interpretable automated coding in clinical practice.

The fourth-ranked team introduced Tumor-RAG, a training-free tumor coding classification method that integrates LLMs with a RAG pipeline. Their approach operates in three stages: extracting pathological staging features from patient records using LLMs, retrieving matching tumor codes from a pre-trained vector database, and reordering these codes via LLMs to determine the final result. The team utilized open-source LLMs, such as ChatGLM-Plus and Qwen-Max, and employed advanced prompt engineering to ensure accurate information extraction and minimal hallucinations. By embedding tumor codes and clinical cases into a vector database and leveraging Faiss for similarity-based retrieval.

The fifth-ranked team developed a medical information extraction and classification framework tailored for lymphoma diagnosis and tumor coding. Their method involves four key stages: preprocessing raw data to align with ICD-10 standards, extracting lymphoma-related information using LLMs, augmenting data via fine-tuning with Chat-GPT and LoRA techniques, and transforming the generative coding task into a classification problem for improved accuracy. By integrating CoT prompting, they ensured stepwise information extraction and classification. The framework classifies diseases into ICD-10 categories and generates ICD-O-M and ICD-O-H codes, addressing challenges in generative tasks by refining the model's outputs with structured options.

5 Conclusion

This paper presents an overview of the "Lymphoma Information Extraction and Automatic Coding Task" organized by CHIP 2024, which focused on evaluating large language models (LLMs) for accurate tumor registry coding. It covers the task design, dataset description, evaluation metrics, and the innovative methodologies employed by the top-performing teams. The dataset and coding task provided a comprehensive testbed for automated ICD-10 and ICD-O-3 coding, pushing the boundaries of LLM application in clinical informatics. In the future, researchers can leverage this dataset to explore novel algorithms or enhance LLMs for broader applications in medical coding and clinical decision support systems.

Acknowledgement. This work was supported by the National Social Science Fund of China (grant number 72274139).

References

1. Kuppers, R., Duhrsen, U., Hansmann, M.L.: Pathogenesis, diagnosis, and treatment of composite lymphomas. Lancet Oncol. **15**(10), e435-46 (2014)
2. Brice, P., de Kerviler, E., Friedberg, J.W.: Classical Hodgkin lymphoma. Lancet **398**(10310), 1518–1527 (2021)
3. Armitage, J.O., et al.: Non-Hodgkin lymphoma. Lancet **390**(10091), 298–310 (2017)
4. Dong, H., et al.: Automated clinical coding: what, why, and where we are? NPJ Digit. Med. **5**(1), 159 (2022)
5. Zong, H., et al.: Large Language Models in Worldwide Medical Exams: Platform Development and Comprehensive Analysis. J. Med. Internet Res. **26**, e66114 (2024)
6. Zong, H., et al.: Advancing Chinese biomedical text mining with community challenges. J. Biomed. Inform. **157**, 104716 (2024)
7. Zhou, L., et al.: Construction of a semi-automatic ICD-10 coding system. BMC Med. Inform. Decis. Mak. **20**(1), 67 (2020)
8. Farkas, R., Szarvas, G.: Automatic construction of rule-based ICD-9-CM coding systems. BMC Bioinform. **9**(Suppl. 3), S10 (2008)

9. Friedman, C., et al.: Automated encoding of clinical documents based on natural language processing. J. Am. Med. Inform. Assoc. **11**(5), 392–402 (2004)

10. Chen, Y., Lu, H., Li, L.: Automatic ICD-10 coding algorithm using an improved longest common subsequence based on semantic similarity. PLoS ONE **12**(3), e0173410 (2017)

11. Chen, P.F., et al.: Automatic ICD-10 coding and training system: deep neural network based on supervised learning. JMIR Med. Inform. **9**(8), e23230 (2021)

12. Li, M., et al.: Automated ICD-9 coding via a deep learning approach. IEEE/ACM Trans. Comput. Biol. Bioinform. **16**(4), 1193–1202 (2019)

13. Yu, Y., et al.: Automatic ICD code assignment of Chinese clinical notes based on multilayer attention BiRNN. J. Biomed. Inform. **91**, 103114 (2019)

14. Farrell, S., et al.: PetBERT: automated ICD-11 syndromic disease coding for outbreak detection in first opinion veterinary electronic health records. Sci. Rep. **13**(1), 18015 (2023)

15. Li, X., et al.: Automatic international classification of diseases coding via note-code interaction network with denoising mechanism. J. Comput. Biol. **30**(8), 912–925 (2023)

16. Ong, J., et al.: Applying large language model artificial intelligence for retina international classification of diseases (ICD) coding. J. Med. Artif. Intell. **6** (2023)

17. Suvirat, K., et al.: Leveraging language models for inpatient diagnosis coding. Appl. Sci. **13**(16), 9450 (2023)

18. Soroush, A., et al.: Large language models are poor medical coders—benchmarking of medical code querying. NEJM AI **1**(5), AIdbp2300040 (2024)

Automatic ICD Code Generation for Lymphoma Using Large Language Models

Yu Song[1], Bohan Yu[1], Pe ngcheng Wu[1], Wenhui Fu[1], Xia Liu[1], Chenxin Hu[2], Kunli Zhang[1(✉)], and Hongying Zan[1]

[1] School of Computer Science and Artificial Intelligence, Zhengzhou University, 450001 Zhengzhou, China
ieklzhang@zzu.edu.cn
[2] Department of Information Science, Affiliated Cancer Hospital of Zhengzhou University (Henan Cancer Hospital), 450000 Zhengzhou, China

Abstract. Lymphoma is a malignant tumor originating from the lymphatic system, with a high global incidence. However, due to the numerous subtypes of lymphoma, each with unique clinical features and diagnostic criteria, accurately coding lymphoma remains challenging. This paper proposes a method for automatically generating ICD codes using large language models. By introducing Automatic Prompt Engineering (APE), we enable the model to generate high-quality prompts autonomously. We further break down the automatic coding process into three stages: disease diagnosis, disease matching, and disease mapping, and apply reasoning and action steps within the Reasoning and Act (ReAct) framework. Our method has shown excellent results across ICD-10, ICD-O-M, and ICD-O-H, ultimately ranking first with a comprehensive score of 92.96%.

Keywords: Large Language Models · Lymphoma · Natural Language Processing

1 Introduction

In the diagnosis and treatment of lymphoma, the International Classification of Diseases (ICD) coding plays a crucial role. It provides a standardized classification for lymphoma and its various subtypes, assisting healthcare professionals worldwide in accurately and consistently recording and communicating disease information. The ICD system assigns a unique code to each lymphoma subtype, ensuring precise clinical treatment planning and providing reliable data support for disease statistics and epidemiological research.

With the exponential growth of medical data, traditional manual coding methods are no longer sufficient to meet the demands for efficiency and accuracy. As a result, ICD automatic coding systems have become an important research direction in the field of medical informatics. Traditional ICD coding relies on

© The Author(s), under exclusive license to Springer Nature Singapore Pte Ltd. 2025
Y. Zhang et al. (Eds.): CHIP 2024, CCIS 2458, pp. 85–92, 2025.
https://doi.org/10.1007/978-981-96-4298-4_8

expert input and classification, which is inefficient and prone to errors. However, automatic coding methods based on natural language processing (NLP) and deep learning technologies can prarse unstructured text in Electronic Health Records (EHRs), automating and standardizing the coding process, thereby significantly improving efficiency and accuracy.

In this study, we address the automatic coding of lymphoma by utilizing Large Language Models (LLMs) for the automatic construction of ICD codes. We integrate Automatic Prompt Engineering (APE), enabling the model to generate high-quality prompts autonomously. Additionally, within the ReAct framework, we design reasoning and action steps, breaking the automatic coding task into three core components: disease diagnosis, matching, and mapping. Our experiments show that this method achieves excellent performance in ICD-10, ICD-O-M, and ICD-O-H coding tasks, ultimately ranking first with a comprehensive score of 92.96%.

2   Related Work

Early research on ICD code automation primarily relied on rule-based systems and traditional machine learning techniques. Although these methods laid the foundation for automating ICD coding, they typically required extensive feature engineering and had certain limitations [20]. With the rapid development of deep learning, researchers began to treat the ICD coding task as a multi-label classification problem and attempted to solve it using various neural network models. For instance, some studies used multi-filter residual convolutional neural networks to extract features, thus improving the model's performance [2,7,9]. Additionally, dilated convolutional neural networks (Dilated CNNs) were employed to capture more subtle semantic features. Meanwhile, recurrent neural networks were applied to clinical text encoding, yielding promising results [11,14,18].

In recent years, methods based on pre-trained language models have emerged as the new state-of-the-art technology in this field [5,6,12]. To further improve the model's accuracy and robustness, many studies have started integrating external knowledge into the ICD coding task. This external knowledge includes coding label information, synonyms, knowledge graphs, and the hierarchical structure of the ICD system [15,16,18–22,24,25]. Besides traditional classification methods, some studies also applied text similarity and matching techniques to improve ICD coding. For example, some research used the longest common subsequence (LCS) and semantic similarity methods to match doctors' diagnoses with ICD-10 disease descriptions [4]. Furthermore, some studies employed text similarity methods to match standardized ICD codes with text strings [13]. The introduction of deep matching networks has also effectively improved the performance of ICD-10 coding tasks [3,10,26].

Recently, LLMs have made significant breakthroughs in the field of NLP, and due to their powerful language understanding and generation capabilities, they have been widely applied across various tasks. In the medical field, LLMs have sparked great interest among researchers in automating clinical coding. However, early studies indicated that LLMs tend to make errors when generating medical codes, making them unsuitable for direct application in medical coding tasks [17]. To address this issue, some studies have enhanced LLM performance in medical coding by introducing tools and retrieval mechanisms [8]. Inspired by these works, we combined APE with the ReAct framework, further enhancing the performance of LLMs in ICD coding. Our experimental results demonstrate that the proposed method has significantly improved coding accuracy.

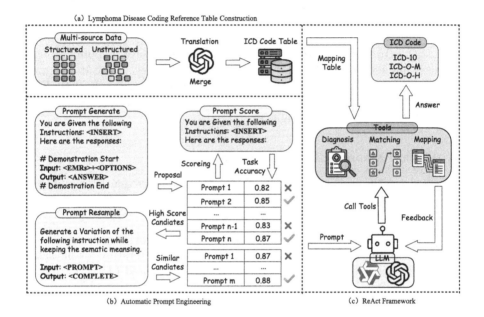

Fig. 1. Overreview of our framework.

3   Method

This section outlines the methods employed, as shown in Fig. 1, which consists of three main stages. In the Disease Code Mapping Table Construction stage, LLMs are used to integrate both structured and unstructured data. Given the presence of English terms, a Chinese-English disease name mapping strategy is adopted to ensure consistent disease name unification across languages. In the APE stage, multiple prompt templates are created to optimize the large language model's responses and result generation. In the ReAct Framework stage, three core steps are defined based on the ReAct framework: Disease Diagnosis, Disease Matching, and Code Mapping. These steps are designed to enhance the model's accuracy and efficiency by ensuring effective disease identification and name mapping.

The disease code mapping table is essential for classifying and coding diseases. It provides standard codes for lymphoma and its subtypes, such as ICD-10

Table 1. Disease code mapping for lymphoma

Disease	ICD-10	ICD-O-M
Malignant lymphoma, NOS	C85.9	9590/3
B-cell lymphoma, NOS	C85.1	9591/3
Primary cutaneous follicle center lymphoma	C85.7	9596/3
(Classical) Hodgkin lymphoma, lymphocyte-rich	C81.4	9651/3
Burkitt cell leukemia	C83.7	9687/3

and ICD-O-3. In this evaluation, we created a comprehensive mapping table to accurately link lymphoma subtypes to their respective codes. To ensure accuracy and coverage, we integrated data from multiple sources, including ICD-10, ICD-O-3, and other national and international classification standards. A sample of the mapping data is shown in Table 1.

3.1   Disease Mapping Table Construction

In constructing the mapping table, we addressed data heterogeneity and diverse sources through two key steps.

Unstructured Data Processing. Some sources provide information in unstructured formats, such as text descriptions, clinical literature, or physician records. To convert this data into structured coding, we used LLMs. LLMs can extract critical information like keywords, diagnostic highlights, and disease categories, accurately mapping them to ICD-10 and ICD-O-3 codes.

Translation and Integration of English Data. Some disease names were in English and needed alignment with Chinese classifications. We implemented a mapping strategy using LLMs for intelligent translation. Beyond simple word substitution, this process included contextual understanding and precise handling of medical terminology. Post-translation, English and Chinese names were cross-verified to ensure semantic equivalence, providing a robust foundation for integration.

3.2   Automatic Prompt Engineering

LLMs demonstrate strong general-purpose capabilities when guided by natural language instructions. However, their performance largely depends on the quality of prompts, which are often manually crafted. Designing effective prompts involves significant trial and error, as small variations can greatly influence the output. In this evaluation, we introduced APE, which aims to identify high-quality prompts from a candidate pool and refine them through exploratory search. APE consists of three main steps.

Generating Candidate Prompts. LLMs are used to create a pool of prompt candidates through two methods: forward mode and reverse mode. In forward mode, task examples are provided first, and the LLM generates prompts at the end. In reverse mode, the target prompt is placed before the examples, and the LLM completes the prompt using a fill-in-the-blank approach.

Selecting High-Quality Prompts. Given the large size of the original training set, we first evaluate the prompts on a small subset, filtering out low-quality ones. This process is repeated iteratively until the candidate pool is sufficiently reduced, at which point the remaining prompts are evaluated on the full training set to identify the highest-scoring prompts.

Sampling High-Quality Prompts. Based on the high-quality prompts identified in the previous step, we use the LLM to sample additional prompts with similar semantics. These sampled prompts are added back to the candidate pool, and the selection process is repeated.

3.3 ReAct

ReAct is a framework designed to improve the performance of intelligent agents in dynamic environments by integrating reasoning and action. It emphasizes that agents should not only perform actions but also reason before each step to enable more flexible and effective decision-making. The framework consists of two key processes.

Reasoning. Helps the agent understand the current environment and generate potential action plans. Using LLMs (e.g., GPT-4o [1], Qwen2.5-72B-Instruct [23]), the agent analyzes complex tasks and environmental features to provide diverse interpretations and strategies.

Act. Translates reasoning into actions. The agent adjusts its decisions based on real-time feedback, reassessing and refining its strategy to stay aligned with task objectives. If an action fails, the agent re-evaluates and updates its approach accordingly.

4   Experiment

4.1   Dataset

The task aims to extract and classify relevant clinical diagnostic codes from lymphoma case reports. The given case text typically includes basic patient information, examination results, diagnostic process, treatment plan, and follow-up details. The model's objective is to accurately extract the clinical diagnostic codes based on this text.

This evaluation task is divided into two parts: the A leaderboard and the B leaderboard. The training set contains 54 data samples, and both the A and B leaderboard test sets also consist of 54 data samples. All data are sourced from published Chinese medical clinical case reports. During the model performance evaluation, the assessment includes three parts: ICD-10, ICD-O-M, and ICD-O-H. The weights for these three parts are 0.3, 0.5, and 0.2, respectively. The final model score will be calculated using the Eq. 1:

$$Acc = 0.3 * Acc_{ICD-10} + 0.5 * Acc_{ICD-O-M} + 0.2 * Acc_{ICD-O-H} \quad (1)$$

4.2 Experimental Setup

In this evaluation, we utilized two large language models, Qwen2.5-72B-Instruct and GPT-4o, to process the task. The parameters for the models' generation are shown in Table 2.

Table 2. Hyperparameter Settings

Hyperparameter	Value
Max_Tokens	2048 (Data Cleaning)/64 (Diagnosis, Matching)
Temperature	0.8
Top-P	0.7
Top-K	50

Table 3. Model Performance

Model	ICD-O-M	ICD-10	ICD-O-H	Overall
Qwen2.5-72B-Instruct	88.89	85.19	94.44	88.88
GPT-4o	92.59	92.59	94.44	92.96

4.3 Experiment Result

Table 3 shows the performance of our method across all subtasks on the B leaderboard test set. As illustrated in the table, our approach achieved strong results in each subtask, with the model's performance having a noticeable impact on individual subtask outcomes. Notably, in the initial diagnosis and disease mapping tasks, GPT-4o significantly outperformed Qwen2.5-72B-Instruct, demonstrating higher accuracy. Ultimately, our method achieved an overall score of 92.96% on the B leaderboard test set, highlighting the model's efficiency and accuracy.

The model, despite achieving a high overall score, exhibited issues such as misclassifications caused by ambiguous or complex clinical language, inconsistent Chinese-English disease naming leading to mapping errors, and sensitivity to low-quality prompts generated by the APE framework. Additionally, noise in EMRs, such as irrelevant or redundant information, further distracted the model from focusing on key diagnostic elements. Addressing these issues through enhanced mapping strategies, improved prompt generation, and noise-filtering mechanisms could significantly improve performance.

5 Conclusion

In this evaluation, we proposed an automated lymphoma ICD coding method based on large language models, integrating the APE and ReAct frameworks to effectively enhance coding accuracy and robustness. By automatically generating high-quality prompts and breaking down the coding task into three steps-disease diagnosis, matching, and mapping—we significantly improved the efficiency and accuracy of traditional ICD coding methods when handling complex medical data. Experimental results demonstrate that the proposed method performed exceptionally well across ICD-10, ICD-O-M, and ICD-O-H coding tasks, achieving the top overall score of 92.96%, underscoring its potential in automated medical coding.

Acknowledgments. The Science and Technology Innovation 2030–"New Generation of Artificial Intelligence" Major Project [No. 2021ZD0111000], and Henan Provincial Science and Technology Research Project [No. 232102211033].

References

1. Achiam, J., et al.: GPT-4 technical report (2023). arXiv preprint arXiv:2303.08774
2. Cao, P., et al.: Clinical-coder: assigning interpretable ICD-10 codes to Chinese clinical notes. In: Proceedings of the 58th Annual Meeting of the Association for Computational Linguistics: System Demonstrations, pp. 294–301 (2020)
3. Chen, Y., Chen, H., Lu, X., Duan, H., He, S., An, J.: Automatic ICD-10 coding: deep semantic matching based on analogical reasoning. Heliyon **9**(4) (2023)
4. Chen, Y., Lu, H., Li, L.: Automatic ICD-10 coding algorithm using an improved longest common subsequence based on semantic similarity. PloS One **12**(3), e0173410 (2017)
5. Coutinho, I., Martins, B.: Transformer-based models for ICD-10 coding of death certificates with Portuguese text. J. Biomed. Inform. **136**, 104232 (2022)
6. Huang, C.W., Tsai, S.C., Chen, Y.N.: PLM-ICD: automatic ICD coding with pre-trained language models. In: Proceedings of the 4th Clinical Natural Language Processing Workshop, pp. 10–20 (2022)
7. Ji, S., Pan, S., Marttinen, P.: Medical code assignment with gated convolution and note-code interaction. In: Findings of the Association for Computational Linguistics: ACL-IJCNLP 2021, pp. 1034–1043 (2021)
8. Kwan, K.: Large language models are good medical coders, if provided with tools (2024). arXiv preprint arXiv:2407.12849
9. Li, F., Yu, H.: ICD coding from clinical text using multi-filter residual convolutional neural network. In: Proceedings of the AAAI Conference on Artificial Intelligence, vol. 34, pp. 8180–8187 (2020)

10. Mou, C., Ren, J.: Automated ICD-10 code assignment of nonstandard diagnoses via a two-stage framework. Artif. Intell. Med. **108**, 101939 (2020)
11. Mullenbach, J., Wiegreffe, S., Duke, J., Sun, J., Eisenstein, J.: Explainable prediction of medical codes from clinical text. In: Proceedings of the 2018 Conference of the North American Chapter of the Association for Computational Linguistics: Human Language Technologies, Volume 1 (Long Papers), pp. 1101–1111 (2018)
12. Pascual, D., Luck, S., Wattenhofer, R.: Towards BERT-based automatic ICD coding: limitations and opportunities. In: Proceedings of the 20th Workshop on Biomedical Language Processing, pp. 54–63 (2021)
13. Pérez, A., Atutxa, A., Casillas, A., Gojenola, K., Sellart, Á.: Inferred joint multigram models for medical term normalization according to ICD. Int. J. Med. Inform. **110**, 111–117 (2018)
14. Shi, H., Xie, P., Hu, Z., Zhang, M., Xing, E.P.: Towards automated ICD coding using deep learning (2017). arXiv preprint arXiv:1711.04075
15. Sonabend, A., et al.: Automated ICD coding via unsupervised knowledge integration (unite). Int. J. Med. Inform. **139**, 104135 (2020)
16. Song, C., Zhang, S., Sadoughi, N., Xie, P., Xing, E.: Generalized zero-shot text classification for ICD coding. In: Proceedings of the Twenty-Ninth International Conference on International Joint Conferences on Artificial Intelligence, pp. 4018–4024 (2021)
17. Soroush, A., et al.: Large language models are poor medical coders-benchmarking of medical code querying. NEJM AI **1**(5), AIdbp2300040 (2024)
18. Vu, T., Nguyen, D.Q., Nguyen, A.: A label attention model for ICD coding from clinical text. In: Proceedings of the Twenty-Ninth International Conference on International Joint Conferences on Artificial Intelligence, pp. 3335–3341 (2021)
19. Wang, G., et al.: Joint embedding of words and labels for text classification. In: Proceedings of the 56th Annual Meeting of the Association for Computational Linguistics (Volume 1: Long Papers), pp. 2321–2331 (2018)
20. Wu, Y., Zeng, M., Fei, Z., Yu, Y., Wu, F.X., Li, M.: KAICD: a knowledge attention-based deep learning framework for automatic ICD coding. Neurocomputing **469**, 376–383 (2022)
21. Xie, X., Xiong, Y., Yu, P.S., Zhu, Y.: EHR coding with multi-scale feature attention and structured knowledge graph propagation. In: Proceedings of the 28th ACM International Conference on Information and Knowledge Management, pp. 649–658 (2019)
22. Yan, J., et al.: Text2tree: aligning text representation to the label tree hierarchy for imbalanced medical classification. In: Findings of the Association for Computational Linguistics: EMNLP 2023, pp. 7705–7720 (2023)
23. Yang, A., et al.: Qwen2 technical report (2024). arXiv preprint arXiv:2407.10671
24. Yu, Y., Duan, J., Jiang, H., Wang, J.: Automatic ICD coding based on multigranularity feature fusion. In: International Symposium on Bioinformatics Research and Applications, pp. 19–29. Springer, Cham (2022)
25. Yuan, Z., Tan, C., Huang, S.: Code synonyms do matter: multiple synonyms matching network for automatic ICD coding. In: Proceedings of the 60th Annual Meeting of the Association for Computational Linguistics (Volume 2: Short Papers), pp. 808–814 (2022)
26. Zong, H., et al.: Advancing Chinese biomedical text mining with community challenges. J. Biomed. Inform. 104716 (2024)

Lymphoma Tumor Coding and Information Extraction: A Comparative Analysis of Large Language Model-Based Methods

Jian Hou[1], Fen Yang[2], Weihua Chen[1], Yining Wang[1], Jing Feng[1], Jin Shi[1], Jiahui Fan[1], Jianlin Li[2(✉)], Jinmin Gu[2], Siyu Lv[2], and Yingying Cen[2]

[1] Unisound AI Technology Co. Ltd., Beijing 100096, China
[2] The Eighth Affiliated Hospital, Sun Yat-sen University, Shenzhen 518033, China
Jianlin66@126.com

Abstract. This study addresses the challenges of information extraction and complete tumor registry coding for lymphoma [1], a malignancy originating from the lymphatic system. Lymphoma encompasses various subtypes, primarily classified into Hodgkin lymphoma and non-Hodgkin lymphoma, both of which exhibit a high incidence globally. Accurate coding of lymphoma diagnoses is particularly challenging due to the complexity and diversity of its subtypes, each possessing unique clinical features and diagnostic criteria. The research explores the potential of large language models (LLMs) in automating the coding process for lymphoma clinical diagnoses by leveraging extensive medical literature, case reports, and clinical guidelines. By simulating the cognitive processes of human coders, these models can offer personalized coding suggestions, thereby enhancing the accuracy and efficiency of diagnostic coding. Through a comparative analysis of coding results generated by LLMs and human coders, this study aims to evaluate the strengths and limitations of these models, ultimately promoting their application in clinical practice. We employed a pipeline with lymphoma info extraction, GraphRAG, and mutual mapping for accuracy enhancement. Our UniGPT model, trained on bilingual and medical data, was assessed for effectiveness.

Keywords: Large Language Model (LLM) · Lymphoma diagnose · Information Extraction · GraphRAG

1 Introduction

Lymphoma, a type of cancer that arises from the lymphatic system, represents a significant public health concern due to its increasing prevalence worldwide. It is primarily categorized into two major types: Hodgkin lymphoma and non-Hodgkin lymphoma, each with distinct clinical characteristics and treatment

---

J. Hou and F. Yang—These authors contributed equally to this work.

© The Author(s), under exclusive license to Springer Nature Singapore Pte Ltd. 2025
Y. Zhang et al. (Eds.): CHIP 2024, CCIS 2458, pp. 93–102, 2025.
https://doi.org/10.1007/978-981-96-4298-4_9

protocols. The complexity of lymphoma diagnosis necessitates a comprehensive evaluation of various clinical data, including patient history, physical examinations, laboratory tests, imaging studies, and particularly, pathological assessments. The accurate coding of these diagnoses is crucial for effective patient management, epidemiological studies, and healthcare resource allocation.

Clinical diagnostic coding serves as a vital mechanism for transforming intricate clinical information into standardized codes, facilitating the systematic recording and analysis of medical data [2,3]. However, the task of generating complete tumor registry codes for lymphoma is fraught with challenges due to the multitude of lymphoma subtypes and their respective diagnostic criteria. This complexity underscores the need for innovative solutions to enhance the accuracy and efficiency of coding practices.

Recent years, the impact of large language models (LLMs) like GPT on medical field and healthcare is growing, which becomes an innovation power for medical treatment [4]. In this research, we investigated the application of LLMs to automate the coding process. Our approach involved a pipeline that included extracting lymphoma information through prompt engineering and GraphRAG (Fig. 1), utilizing a coarse-to-fine ranking method for encoding retrieval, and applying mutual mapping for post-processing, all aimed at improving coding accuracy. We employed our large language model, UniGPT, which was trained on a significant amount of bilingual data and further refined with medical data, and we assessed the effectiveness of our method [7–10].

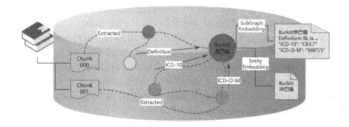

Fig. 1. The Process of Constructing Medical Knowledge Graph.

2   Related Work

2.1   Prompt Engineering

Prompt engineering [11,12] has emerged as a vital technique for effectively interacting with large language models (LLMs) in the context of their widespread application. This approach involves the design and refinement of prompts, instructions given to AI models, which can range from simple questions and textual materials to more complex inputs like images, audio, or video clips. The goal of prompt engineering is to enhance the performance of LLMs, creating systems that are both effective and controllable, enabling them to accurately and reliably carry out specific tasks [13,14].

The prompts suggested by researchers such as Timo et al. demonstrate the versatility of this method in handling various natural language processing (NLP) tasks. However, successful implementation requires careful cue engineering, either through manual crafting or automated processes, since LLMs do not interpret cues with the same nuanced understanding as humans. Liu et al. have introduced efficient fast-tuning techniques using gradient-based optimization methods, yet the computational cost of calculating gradients presents challenges, especially when accessing models via APIs that may not allow gradient access, complicating scalability [15].

Prompt engineering can be categorized into three distinct types: zero-shot learning, where models classify previously unseen categories to exhibit reasoning akin to human intelligence; one-shot learning, which involves training with only a single example of each category; and few-shot learning, where a limited number of examples are used during training to guide the model's predictions on new tasks. Overall, prompt engineering represents a critical intersection of artificial intelligence and human intuition, aimed at optimizing how LLMs perform across diverse applications [16].

2.2 Embedding

In the field of natural language processing (NLP), large language models (LLMs) are powerful tools capable of generating and summarizing text. However, a lesser-known aspect of these models lies in their ability to create embeddings. These embeddings are numerical representations of words within a multi-dimensional space, capturing the essence of language in a quantifiable manner. LLMs utilize their deep understanding of language to generate embeddings that encode complex semantic and syntactic relationships. This goes beyond simply producing text; it allows us to capture the nuances, subtleties, and hidden connections within language itself [17].

To efficiently store these embeddings, vector databases are employed. Unlike traditional databases which rely on rows and columns, vector databases use algorithms to index these numerical representations. They search for the most similar vector to a given query using function approximation, a process known as Retrieval Augmented Generation (RAG). RAG enhances LLM responses by supplementing their context beyond their training data.

In essence, embeddings allow us to bridge the gap between human language and machine understanding. They offer a powerful tool for analyzing and manipulating language, enabling LLMs to go beyond simply generating text and unlock a deeper, more nuanced understanding of the world [18].

2.3 Tumor Coding

Coding Purpose: Tumor types, typically represented as codes, are crucial for the organized management of medical information. The use of coding systems such as the International Classification of Diseases for Oncology (ICD-O) is essential for cancer registries, clinical trials, and epidemiological research [5].

Application in Healthcare: In electronic health records, standardized coding promotes effective data management and analysis. For disease surveillance, it assists in monitoring the occurrence and distribution of various cancer types. In research, consistent nomenclature and coding are vital for accurate data collection and comparison across different studies [6].

Importance of Standardization: The necessity of standardizing tumor nomenclature and coding improve the quality of healthcare data. This standardization ensures accurate information capture, minimizing the risk of errors and misunderstandings. It also facilitates data sharing among various healthcare systems and countries, which is especially important for global health initiatives and collaborative research projects.

3 Methodology

3.1 Datasets

The dataset is composed of published Chinese medical clinical case reports. Through screening, 162 case reports related to lymphoma were identified. Among them, there are 54 cases in the training set, 54 cases in test set A, and 54 cases in test set B.

Overview of the generation scheme: To create an effective generation scheme, we need to clearly define the input (the patient's textual information) and the output (the content the model needs to generate), and also set some rules to ensure that the generated content is accurate, useful, and meets standards. The goal is, by inputting the patient's basic information, the model should be able to generate the corresponding clinical diagnostic codes.

Input format: Patient information (text): The text generally includes information such as the patient's basic data, examinations, diagnoses, and treatments. For example: Diffuse large B-cell lymphoma (DLBCL) is a type that originates from organs.

3.2 Pipeline

In this competition, we implemented our approach in three steps: lymphoma information extraction, encoding retrieval, and post-processing. The whole pipeline is shown as Fig. 2.

The first step is lymphoma information extraction. We utilized our self-developed medical large language model to extract pathological staging information from case reports related to lymphoma. Since the competition provided 54 data entries, we realized that training on this data directly would not yield good results. Therefore, we employed prompt engineering combined with the RAG (Retrieval-Augmented Generation) approach, introducing GraphRAG to structurally process the text and provide the corresponding extraction results.

The second step involves encoding retrieval of the extracted results. We adopted a coarse-to-fine ranking method for retrieval, using keyword and semantic vector search to match the output tumor staging from the medical records with those in our database.

In the third step, during the post-processing phase, we performed a mutual mapping. This process stemmed from our observation that many ICD-10 codes in the ICD table contain ICD-O-M codes, and some ICD-O-M codes include ICD-10 codes. We found that this mapping could improve the accuracy of the coding.

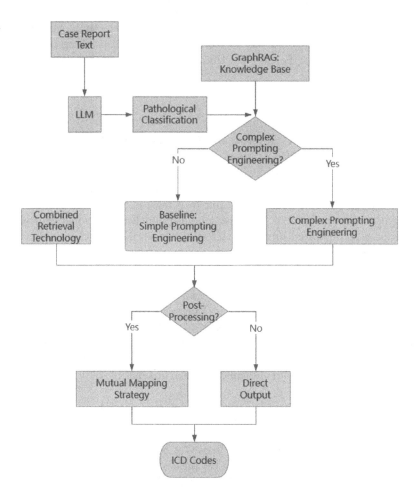

Fig. 2. GraphRAG workflow shows the whole process of generating ICD codes.

3.3 Multi-vec Retrieval

Multi-Vec Retrieval is a text retrieval technique based on vector representation. The fundamental idea is to convert text into vectors in a multi-dimensional space and then retrieve relevant texts by calculating the similarity between vectors. Specifically, for a given text, we first obtain the hidden states from all positions in the last layer of the language model. These hidden states can be transformed and normalized through a fully connected matrix to obtain the multi-vector representation of the text, with dimensions $n*d$, where n is the length of the text and d is the dimension of the hidden states.

Given a query, we calculate the similarity between the i-th position of the query and the document (doc). This is achieved by calculating the dot product between the multi-vector representation of the i-th position of the query and the multi-vector representations of all positions in the doc. We take the maximum value of these dot products as the score, and then average the similarities between all positions of the query and the doc to obtain the corresponding multi-vector representation similarity. Essentially, this is an extension of dense retrieval.

4 Experiments

4.1 Datasets

Our large model, UniGPT, is based on the Transformer decoder architecture, consisting of 76 layers, with a hidden layer size of 8192, 64 heads, and a total parameter count of 70 billion, which is a gerenalized medical large language model. The size of training data the competition provided is too small to use (54 datapoints), thus we constructed our own dataset without these data. The training data is composed of bilingual Chinese and English, sourced from web scraping and accumulated business data from Unisound Ltd. Company.

4.2 Model and Experimental Setting

Our large model was trained for two months on the Unisound Ltd. Company's proprietary Atlas cluster using our self-developed UniScale framework. To further enhance its medical capabilities, we conducted incremental training using a substantial amount of industry-related data accumulated by Unisound Ltd. Company over many years in the medical field. This data includes medical literature, medical textbooks, and clinical case data, ultimately resulting in a medical large language model.

4.3 Results

For Track B, UniGPT-Med is ranked 2nd. Our team is a collaboration between UniSonund and The Eighth Affiliated Hospital at Sun Yat-sen University, with an average score of 0.9222 (Table 1). The current LLM models which are capable of achieving a level of over 90, indicate a great potential for coding. However, the test set only contains 54 cases, and it is necessary to verify the effectiveness on a larger set.

Table 1. The winning teams and their test results of Track B.

Team Name	Rank	Institution	Avg. Score
PhD.Yu	1	Zhengzhou University (郑州大学)	0.9296
UniGPT-Med	2	UniSound (云知声) and 深圳中大八院	0.9222
大香蕉	3	Hohai University (河海大学)	0.8963
魔法猫	1	Xiangtan University (湘潭大学)	0.8926

5 Evaluation

5.1 Effectiveness of the Baseline Method

The baseline model, GraphRAG, demonstrated an initial performance score of 0.6574 in the ICD coding task. This score serves as a benchmark for subsequent improvements, indicating that the model can achieve a certain level of coding accuracy even without additional optimization. However, it also highlights significant potential for enhancement.

5.2 Impact of Prompt Engineering

The introduction of "prompt engineering" led to a substantial improvement in model performance, with the score increasing from 0.6574 to 0.813. This underscores the critical role that well-designed prompts play in guiding the model to perform better on specific tasks. Prompt engineering aids the model in comprehending context more effectively, thereby enhancing coding precision, particularly in the classifications of ICD-10 and ICD-O-M. This improvement reflects an enhanced understanding of specialized terminology within the professional domain.

5.3 Benefits of Incorporating a Retrieval Mechanism

The integration of a retrieval mechanism further boosted the model's performance, raising the score to 0.8667. This indicates that leveraging precise external knowledge bases or historical cases can significantly enhance the model's decision-making process, especially when dealing with complex or rare disease coding. This not only improves accuracy but also strengthens the model's generalization capabilities.

5.4 Importance of Post-processing

During the stage of post-processing, we adopted bi-directional mapping which could improve the coding accuracy. The reason is we found that code ICD-10 in table ICD might contain code ICD-O-M, and code ICD-O-M might also contain code ICD-10. For instance: The interpretation for ICD-10 code C91.2 is: Subacute Lymphocytic Leukemia 9820/3. It can be observed that when we search for

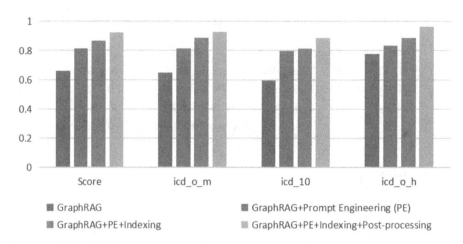

Fig. 3. The impact of different methods (GraphRAG, GraphRAG+Prompt Engineering, GraphRAG+PE+Indexing, GraphRAG+PE+Indexing+Post-processing) on the accuracy of different types of coding (ICD-O-M, ICD-10, ICD-O-H) in the ICD coding task.

the ICD-10 coding table using Subacute Lymphocytic Leukemia, we can simultaneously obtain the ICD-10 code for this disease, as well as its corresponding ICD-O-M code. Therefore, using high-confidence matching results to acquire the final code is a reliable method.

Finally, the implementation of post-processing steps enabled the model to achieve its highest performance score of 0.9222. This finding illustrates that refining the algorithm's outputs is essential for enhancing the accuracy and reliability of the final results. These steps effectively address the shortcomings of the model's predictions, ensuring that the coding adheres strictly to established standards, as Fig. 3.

5.5   Comprehensive Benefits of the Integrated Approach

A comprehensive analysis reveals that each improvement builds cumulatively, resulting in a model that efficiently and accurately handles ICD coding tasks through the combination of prompt engineering, retrieval mechanisms, and post-processing. This not only demonstrates the effects of technological layering but also suggests that the integration of multiple technologies is a key strategy for enhancing performance in the field of medical AI.

5.6   Comprehensive Analysis of the Failure Case

The model first extract the pathological staging from the patients' information and then assign codes based on that staging. Thus, accurately extracting the pathological staging is a vital step that connects two processes, and precision in this extraction is critical. "Accurate" in this context means not only identifying the most relevant pathology from various text entries, but also ensuring consistency with the descriptions in the coding table.

During this process, we faced a significant challenge with abbreviations. For example, the input text states: "Intravascular large B-cell lymphoma (IVLBCL) is a rare and clinically aggressive lymphoma characterized by selective tumor cell growth within blood vessels without lymph node involvement..." The model identified the pathological stage as: "IVLBCL, Stage IVB." However, by checking the ICD-10 coding table, we found no code for "IVLBCL," but we did find a code for "intravascular large B-cell lymphoma," which is C83.8. As a temporary solution, we organized the abbreviations of lymphomas manually to replace the pathological staging or the interpretations in the coding table.

6   Conclusion and Future Work

In this study, we focused on lymphoma, a malignancy of the lymphatic system with significant global prevalence and complex subtypes. The accurate coding of lymphoma diagnoses is crucial for patient management and research but challenging due to subtype diversity. We explored the use of large language models (LLMs) to automate the coding process. By implementing a pipeline including lymphoma information extraction with prompt engineering and GraphRAG, encoding retrieval using a coarse-to-fine ranking method, and post-processing with mutual mapping, we aimed to enhance the accuracy of coding. Our large model, UniGPT, was trained on a substantial amount of bilingual data and further fine-tuned with medical data. Through experiments and evaluations (details in the relevant sections), we were able to assess the performance of our approach. This research contributes to understanding the potential of LLMs in lymphoma diagnosis coding and may pave the way for more efficient and accurate coding practices in clinical applications.

There are three main valuable outcomes learned from past challenges: the great quality and diversity of the datasets; the strong relevance of challenge tasks to real-world clinical needs; the active engagement with the research community in various forms [19].

Future research could explore further optimization of prompt design, expansion of the retrieval database, or the application of more advanced post-processing algorithms to achieve even higher accuracy rates. Additionally, investigating the potential applications of these technologies in other medical diagnostic and coding tasks could yield valuable insights and advancements in the field. Furthermore, according to the failure case, two initiatives are: 1. Improving the ability of large language models (LLMs) to recognize abbreviations by training them on extensive medical or relevant texts, enabling them to generate comprehensive responses as per instructions; 2. Feeding patient information and coding tables into LLMs to directly obtain the final codes, which would necessitate that LLMs possess a robust understanding and the capability to encode lengthy texts.

Acknowledgments. The research work described in this paper has been supported by Shenzhen Technology Innovation Fund under Project No. KCXFZ20230731093001002, and we greatly value the support.

References

1. de Leval, L., Jaffe, E.S.: Lymphoma classification. Cancer J. **26**(3), 176–185 (2020)
2. Li, D., et al.: A deep learning diagnostic platform for diffuse large B-cell lymphoma with high accuracy across multiple hospitals. Nat. Commun. **11**(1), 6004 (2020)
3. Vu, T., Nguyen, D.Q., Nguyen, A.: A label attention model for ICD coding from clinical text, arXiv preprint arXiv:2007.06351 (2020)
4. Ng, J., Fu, P.S., Zhang, R., Phan, K.Y.: The impact and acceptance of large language models in healthcare: a perspective from China. J. Adv. Res. Appl. Sci. Eng. Technol. 110–158 (2024)
5. Kaur, R., Ginige, J.A., Obst, O.: AI-based ICD coding and classification approaches using discharge summaries: a systematic literature review. Expert Syst. Appl. **213**, 118997 (2023)
6. Walls, M., et al.: Developmental-behavioral pediatricians' diagnosis and coding of overweight and obesity in children with autism Spectrum disorder. J. Dev. Behav. Pediatr. **41**(4), 258–264 (2020)
7. Wu, J., Zhu, J., Qi, Y.: Medical graph rag: towards safe medical large language model via graph retrieval-augmented generation, arXiv preprint arXiv:2408.04187 (2024)
8. Magham, R.K.: Graphrag and role of graph databases in advancing AI. Int. J. Res. Comput. Appl. Inf. Technol. (IJRCAIT) **7**(2), 98–110 (2024)
9. Hu, Y., et al.: GRAG: Graph Retrieval-Augmented Generation, arXiv preprint arXiv:2405.16506 (2024)
10. Yang, R., et al.: Graphusion: A RAG Framework for Knowledge Graph Construction with a Global Perspective, arXiv preprint arXiv:2410.17600 (2024)
11. Mesko, B.: Prompt engineering as an important emerging skill for medical professionals: tutorial. J. Med. Internet Res. **25**, e50638 (2023)
12. Chen, B., et al.: Unleashing the potential of prompt engineering in Large Language Models: a comprehensive review, arXiv preprint arXiv:2310.14735 (2023)
13. Wang, J., et al.: Prompt engineering for healthcare: methodologies and applications, arXiv preprint arXiv:2304.14670 (2023)
14. Patil, R., et al.: Prompt engineering in healthcare. Electronics **13**(15), 2961 (2024)
15. Sahoo, P., et al.: A systematic survey of prompt engineering in large language models: techniques and applications, arXiv preprint arXiv:2402.07927 (2024)
16. Zhou, Y., et al.: Large language models are human-level prompt engineers, arXiv preprint arXiv:2211.01910 (2022)
17. Hu, J., et al.: Enhancing sequential recommendation via LLM-based semantic embedding learning. In: Companion Proceedings of the ACM on Web Conference 2024, pp. 103–111 (2024)
18. Peng, R., et al.: Embedding-based retrieval with LLM for effective agriculture information extracting from unstructured data, arXiv preprint arXiv:2308.03107 (2023)
19. Zong, H., et al.: Advancing Chinese biomedical text mining with community challenges. J. Biomed. Inform. **157**, 104716 (2024). https://doi.org/10.1016/j.jbi.2024.104716

Leveraging Chain of Thought for Automated Medical Coding of Lymphoma Cases

Wenlong Song, Jiaxin Hu, Zixuan Li, and Chi Yuan[✉]

College of Computer Science and Software Engineering, Hohai University,
Nanjing, China
20210021@hhu.edu.cn

Abstract.

Objective: This study aims to explore the application of Chain of Thought (CoT) reasoning in automating ICD coding, specifically focusing on lymphoma cases. By leveraging large language models (LLMs) and CoT prompting, the research aims to improve the accuracy and interpretability of automated ICD coding in healthcare.

Methods: We optimized CoT prompting for Qwen 2.5:14b to guide the model in reasoning through the diagnostic process in a step-by-step manner. There are three main components for our pipeline. This framework was then evaluated on multiple LLMs, including Qwen 2.5, Llama 3.1, and Gemma 2, using a clinical lymphoma dataset for automated ICD-10 and ICD-O coding tasks. The models were assessed on their ability to extract relevant diagnoses from clinical text and map them to appropriate ICD codes.

Results: The results indicated that CoT reasoning improves the interpretability and accuracy of ICD coding. However, the generalizability of CoT-based prompt design is not guaranteed for all the LLMs. Prompts optimized for one model do not consistently transfer to others, highlighting the importance of customizing prompts for each specific model.

Conclusion: Our findings suggest that CoT reasoning can enhance automated ICD coding when tailored to the characteristics of each model. Future work should focus on optimizing CoT prompting techniques for different models to enhance generalizability and improve the scalability of automated coding systems in healthcare.

1 Introduction

Recent advancements in Artificial Intelligence (AI) have created significant opportunities for the development of smart healthcare systems [1]. Among these advancements, automated medical coding plays a crucial role in enhancing the efficiency and accuracy of healthcare processes. The International Classification of Diseases (ICD), maintained by the World Health Organization (WHO), is a globally recognized classification system for categorizing and coding diseases, injuries, and causes of death [2]. It provides a standardized language for

© The Author(s), under exclusive license to Springer Nature Singapore Pte Ltd. 2025
Y. Zhang et al. (Eds.): CHIP 2024, CCIS 2458, pp. 103–116, 2025.
https://doi.org/10.1007/978-981-96-4298-4_10

healthcare professionals, researchers, and policymakers worldwide, facilitating communication, public health monitoring, and global health comparisons [2]. Widely applied in healthcare, research, and policy-making, ICD coding enables accurate diagnosis, consistent documentation, and efficient resource allocation, making it essential for both patient care and population health management [3]. However, manual ICD coding is labor-intensive [4], requiring domain-specific knowledge, which results in high costs and potential inconsistencies in coding practices across different healthcare settings [5]. These challenges highlight the need for automated ICD coding methods, particularly as the volume of health data grows.

The application of large language models (LLMs) such as ChatGPT in automated ICD code generation has shown promising potential in reducing the administrative burden on healthcare providers [6].

Despite significant advancements, automating ICD coding with LLMs remains an challenging task. Medical language is inherently complex, and the ICD's extensive code set requires high accuracy for clinical applications. While preliminary studies have indicate promising results, challenges persist, such as model interpretability, generalization to diverse healthcare settings, and the need for extensive labeled data for model training [7,8]. Current methods also vary in effectiveness, depending on the complexity of cases and the quality of clinical notes, underscoring a gap in the development of robust, scalable ICD coding solutions.

To further enhance the accuracy and interpretability of LLMs in ICD coding, recent approaches have introduced the Chain of Thought (CoT) method [9]. The CoT technique encourages models to generate intermediate reasoning steps, allowing them to process complex information in a sequential and logical manner before arriving at a final decision [9]. This structured approach aligns well with medical coding tasks, where accurate mapping from clinical descriptions to ICD codes often requires a detailed, step-by-step reasoning process. By prompting models to explicitly "think" through each aspect of the clinical information, CoT enhances both the transparency and reliability of the coding output, especially in complex cases.

This study aims to explore the application of LLMs, by utilizing CoT method to implement accurate and efficient coding in healthcare. Building upon recent advancements in natural language processing (NLP) and machine learning, our research contributes to the growing evidence for the feasibility and impact of LLM-based ICD coding systems. Through this approach, we aim to lessen the burden of manual coding, improve accuracy, and enhance healthcare documentation and data analytics in clinical environments.

Our contributions can be summarized as follows:

- We propose a novel application of LLMs with CoT prompting for automated ICD coding. This approach leverages intermediate reasoning steps to enhance accuracy and interpretability in the coding process, addressing the complexity inherent in medical documentation.
- We design an innovative method that integrates CoT prompting with a knowledge base, enhancing the reasoning capability of LLMs by incorporating struc-

tured domain-specific knowledge into the ICD coding process. This approach improves both the accuracy and interpretability of the model's predictions.

2 Related Work

2.1 Applications of LLMs in Medical Domain

LLMs refer to pre-trained language models (PLMs) of substantial size, typically containing tens to hundreds of billions of parameters. The development of LLMs, such as GPT-3 [10] and GPT-4 [11], has marked a significant advancement in the field, with notable applications like OpenAI's ChatGPT capturing widespread attention. These models not only achieve high performance but also exhibit human-like conversational abilities, influencing both academic research and real-world applications.

Building on these advancements, there has been growing interest in adapting general-purpose LLMs to the medical domain, leading to the emergence of specialized medical LLMs. For example, MedPaLM [12] and MedPaLM-2 [13], based on PaLM, have achieved competitive performance on the United States Medical Licensing Examination (USMLE) [14], with an accuracy of 86.5%, closely matching human expert performance (87.0%). Other medical LLMs, such as ChatDoctor [15], MedAlpaca [16], and PMC-LLaMA [17], have been introduced, based on models like LLaMA.

These medical LLMs are increasingly being explored for their potential to assist healthcare professionals in improving diagnosis, patient care, and medical research, underscoring their growing significance in the healthcare sector. In this study, we leverage Qwen2.5:14b to address the task of automated ICD coding, demonstrating the application of advanced LLMs in healthcare-related tasks.

2.2 Chain of Thought Prompting

CoT prompting has emerged as a promising approach to enhance the reasoning abilities of LLMs, particularly for complex tasks that require multi-step logical or arithmetic reasoning. While prompt engineering has been shown to improve in-context learning by designing more effective prompt templates, LLMs still struggle with intricate reasoning tasks, such as logical inference and arithmetic problems, especially when presented in complex statements.

Wei et al. [9] demonstrated that guiding LLMs through a series of intermediate reasoning steps, referred to as CoT prompting, can significantly enhance their performance on challenging tasks. The simplest approach to CoT is to prompt LLMs with a phrase like "Let's think step by step" [18], encouraging them to articulate their reasoning process before generating the final answer. This zero-shot CoT approach has proven effective in a variety of domains, leading to improved reasoning and prediction accuracy.

CoT prompting has been successfully applied across a range of tasks, including programming [19,20], solving math problems [21], and multi-modal question answering [22], showcasing its versatility in addressing complex, multi-step reasoning challenges. Given this, it is crucial to recognize that automatic ICD coding is a complex reasoning task. In this work, we apply CoT reasoning to support automated ICD coding process, aiming to improve the accuracy and interpretability of the model's coding decisions.

2.3   Automated ICD Coding

Traditional ICD coding has largely relied on manual processes, where trained coders review clinical notes to assign the most relevant codes. This manual coding process, however, is labor-intensive, time-consuming, and subject to inconsistencies, especially as the volume of healthcare data continues to grow [4]. To address these challenges, automated ICD coding has gained research interest, primarily leveraging NLP and machine learning techniques to enhance coding accuracy and efficiency.

Early approaches in automated ICD coding used rule-based [23] and statistical methods, focusing on keyword matching, regular expressions, and simple probabilistic models. While these methods provided initial automation, they often struggled to capture complex medical language and context in clinical notes, limiting their effectiveness. With advancements in machine learning, researchers began applying supervised learning techniques, treating ICD coding as a multi-class, multi-label classification problem. Methods based on support vector machines (SVM), logistic regression, and decision trees demonstrated moderate success but still required extensive feature engineering and failed to generalize well to diverse clinical environments [5].

The application of LLMs to ICD coding has attracted considerable attention in recent years, primarily due to their advanced NLP capabilities. Ong et al. [6] demonstrate that ChatGPT, even without feedback mechanisms, can potentially reduce the burden on physicians by generating a selection of relevant ICD codes. LLMs are adept at analyzing unstructured clinical documentation, identifying pertinent medical concepts, and accurately mapping these concepts to the appropriate ICD codes with minimal human intervention.

Despite these advancements, challenges remain in achieving high accuracy and generalizability for ICD coding, especially in diverse healthcare settings. Limitations include the need for large, high-quality annotated datasets [24], the difficulty of interpreting model decisions, and the challenge of ensuring robustness across different clinical contexts. Continued research into domain-specific adaptations of LLMs, improved training methods, and data augmentation techniques will be essential for advancing automated ICD coding.

3   Methods

3.1   Task Description

The automatic coding task in this challenge can be divided into two subtasks. One is the key diagnosis extraction from clinical texts. For instance, "弥漫大B细胞性非霍奇金淋巴瘤累及骨髓IV期(Diffuse large B-cell non-Hodgkin lymphoma involving the bone marrow, stage IV)" are supposed to be extracted from "...三、诊断与鉴别诊断根据上述结果最终诊断: 1. 弥漫大B细胞淋巴瘤IV期...(...III. Diagnosis and Differential Diagnosis: Based on the above results, the final diagnosis is as follows: 1. Diffuse large B-cell lymphoma, stage IV...)". The other one is mapping extracted diagnoses to the corresponding ICD-10 and ICD-O-3 codes. In the scenario of lymphoma-related coding, the ICD-O-H code, which represents cell origin, is relatively straightforward to determine; however, its accuracy is heavily influenced by the quality of information extracted in the first stage. In the above example, the "弥漫大B细胞性非霍奇金淋巴瘤累及骨髓IV期"should be coded with "C83.3(ICD-10)", "9680/3(ICD-O-M)", "6(ICD-O-H)".

3.2 Automated Medical Coding Pipeline

Our study of the automated medical coding method is mainly made up of three modules: 1) prompt-based diagnosis extraction from clinical text; 2) ICD knowledge- base curation; 3) CoT-based method for automatic ICD coding. The pipeline is illustrated as Fig. 1. The diagnosis information is the basis for ICD coding. Hence, we designed a prompt-based diagnosis extraction module for accurate diagnose concept extraction. Though LLMs were trained with various general knowledge, the ICD coding knowledge is seriously lacking. We created a lymphoma-specialized ICD knowledge base for external knowledge support. Considering the interpretability of clinical practice-oriented method, we developed CoT-based method to guide LLMs to code clinical cases as much like human expert as possible. In the following sections of this chapter, we will focus on introducing the specific implementation of each module.

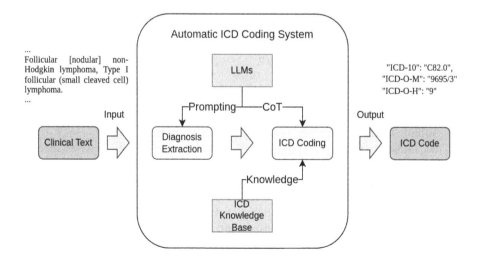

Fig. 1. Automated Medical Coding Pipeline.

3.3   Lymphoma ICD Coding Dataset

The Lymphoma ICD Coding Dataset (LICD), used in this study, was published at the 2024 CHIP conference[1] and is derived from published Chinese
medical clinical case reports. The organizer created a training set consisting of
54 samples, each including textual descriptions and specific diagnostic codes. The
dataset comprises five key attributes, as summarized in Table 1. These attributes
capture both the clinical narrative and the standardized classification of lymphoma cases, offering a comprehensive view of each patient's condition. The
detailed descriptions, along with associated pathological and diagnostic codes,
provide a rich source of information for model training, particularly for automated medical coding tasks. Additionally, two testing sets were published, each
containing 54 samples, and are limited to clinical text only, available to all participants.

Table 1. Key Attributes of the LICD Dataset

Attribute	Description	Example
text	Patient's clinical information	Hemophagocytic syndrome (HPS)...
pathological classification	Diagnoses of the patient.	Diffuse large B-cell non-Hodgkin lymphoma with bone marrow involvement, stage IV
ICD-10	ICD-10 code.	C83.3
ICD-O-M	Histology and behavior code of ICD-O-3 morphology code	9680/3
ICD-O-H	Grading and differentiation level code of ICD-O-3 morphology code	6

3.4   Diagnoses Extraction

As shown in Fig. 2, we utilized a structured prompt design to extract diagnoses
from clinical text using LLMs. The prompt was carefully crafted to guide the
model in identifying and extracting relevant diagnostic information effectively.
It consisted of four essential components:

- **Clinical Text:** A detailed clinical text about a patient.
- **Task Description:** A clear and concise description of the objective to extract
  precise diagnostic details from medical records.
- **Output Format:** A structured format ensuring consistency and clarity in
  the extracted diagnostic data.
- **Example:** A concrete example to demonstrate the expected outputs, enhancing the model's ability to understand and execute the task accurately.

---

[1] http://cips-chip.org.cn/2024/eval2.

Model Input

Clinical Text:

...

Task Description:
You are an expert medical assistant specializing in analyzing clinical records. Your task is to extract diagnoses from the provided clinical text. Focus only on the diagnostic information and exclude unrelated details such as treatments, tests, or general observations.

Output Format:
Return the result as a short phrase. If no diagnosis is identified, respond with "No diagnosis."

Example:
Input: 患者，女性，60岁，因"头晕乏力1个月余，发热1 d"入院。患者1个月前......
       (Patient, female, 60 years old, admitted to the hospital due to "dizziness and fatigue for over 1 month and fever for 1 day." One month ago, the patient...)
Output: 弥漫大B细胞性非霍奇金淋巴瘤累及骨髓IV期
       (Diffuse large B-cell non-Hodgkin lymphoma involving bone marrow, Stage IV)

Fig. 2. Structured prompt for diagnoses extraction. The figure illustrates the three key components: task description, output format, and examples, which collectively ensure effective guidance for the LLM.

The prompt design ensured that the model maintained focus on diagnostic information while adhering to a consistent output structure, resulting in accurate and reliable extractions.

3.5   ICD Knowledge Curation

Explicit curation of ICD-related knowledge for integration with LLMs is essential for several reasons. First, LLMs typically lack domain-specific expertise in medicine, which limits their accuracy and reliability in clinical contexts. Second, LLMs are prone to generating hallucinations—incorrect or misleading information—that can undermine the effectiveness of diagnosis and classification tasks. Lastly, the ICD coding system undergoes periodic updates, making it necessary to continually revise the knowledge base to align with the latest standards in clinical coding and classification.

In the original ICD data, diseases were mapped separately to their corresponding ICD-10 and ICD-O-M codes. To address these challenges, we curated a unified mapping that combines both ICD-10 and ICD-O-M codes for each disease, as represented by the Knowledge in Fig. 3.

3.6   CoT Prompt Construction

To enhance the accuracy and reliability of automated ICD coding, we constructed CoT prompts that imitate the step-by-step reasoning process a human coder would use when assigning codes based on clinical information. By emulating this logical approach, CoT prompts enable LLMs to systematically analyze clinical notes and accurately identify the most relevant ICD codes.

Chain-of-Thought Prompting

Model Input	Model Output
... Follicular [nodular] non-Hodgkin lymphoma, Type I follicular (small cleaved cell) lymphoma. ... Clinical Information: Follicular lymphoma, grade I. Question: Among the given list of codes, which row corresponds to the patient's primary disease (choose only one row)? When the clinical information does not specify a particular subtype, prioritize data entries with "NOS" (not otherwise specified) in the description. Instructions: Follow these steps to determine the answer: Extract the keywords from the clinical information. Search for matching entries in the code list. Finally, provide the answer.	1. Extract the keywords from the clinical information The clinical information provided is: Follicular lymphoma, grade I. From this, we can extract the following keywords: - Follicular - Lymphoma - Grade I 2. Search for matching entries in the code list Based on the extracted keywords, we will search for the most relevant code in the provided code list. Specific subtype information includes grade I, and "Follicular [nodular] non-Hodgkin lymphoma, Type I follicular (small cleaved cell) lymphoma"matches this. Answer: "ICD-10": "C82.0", "ICD-O-M": "9695/3"

Knowledge

- C82.0, 9695/3: Follicular [nodular] non-Hodgkin lymphoma, Type I follicular (small cleaved cell) lymphoma
- C82.1, 9691/3: Follicular [nodular] non-Hodgkin lymphoma, Type II follicular (small cleaved cell and large cell) lymphoma
- C82.2, 9698/3: Follicular [nodular] non-Hodgkin lymphoma, Type III follicular (small cleaved cell and predominantly large cell) lymphoma

Fig. 3. An example of CoT prompt construction for automated ICD coding, illustrating the step-by-step reasoning approach to match clinical information with appropriate codes.

Figure 3 illustrates an example of CoT prompt construction for ICD coding. The process is divided into distinct steps to guide the model through identifying key information, matching it with the matching table, and selecting the most appropriate code. The following steps are demonstrated:

1. **Extract Keywords from Clinical Information:** The model first extracts critical keywords from the clinical information provided. In this example, the clinical data includes terms like "follicular", "lymphoma" and "grade I". From these descriptions, keywords such as "follicular type", "lymphoma", and "grade level" are identified, which will be essential for accurate coding.
2. **Match Keywords with Matching Table:** Using the extracted keywords, the model then searches through the Matching Table to find the most relevant code. As shown in the example, the extracted keywords lead to a match with "follicular lymphoma [nodal] non-Hodgkin lymphoma".
3. **Select the Appropriate Code:** If an exact subtype is not available in the clinical information, the model defaults to selecting a code that includes a general or "NOS" (Not Otherwise Specified) option. This approach mimics human coding decisions, where the coder may choose a broader category if specific details are missing.

The CoT prompts are designed to reflect a logical, human-like reasoning process, improving the interpretability and performance of automated ICD coding systems. By following these structured steps, the model can handle complex cases more effectively, leading to more consistent and accurate coding results.

4 Evaluation

We first optimized the CoT prompt specifically for Qwen2.5:14b to maximize its performance. Subsequently, the same prompt was applied to other LLMs to evaluate their performance under identical conditions, allowing for a comparative analysis of the prompt's effectiveness across different models.

4.1 Large Language Models

Considering the cost of local deployment, our experiments were designed to ensure that the solution is deployable on consumer-grade GPUs. All experiments were conducted on a single NVIDIA RTX 4090, demonstrating that high performance can be achieved with lower hardware costs. This setup ensures that the approach remains accessible to individual researchers and healthcare institutions while maximizing the potential of LLMs.

We evaluated the performance of three LLM families—Llama 3.1, Qwen 2.5, and Gemma 2–on the task of automated ICD coding using the LICD dataset. The evaluation included experiments with and without CoT reasoning to assess its impact on both the accuracy and interpretability of ICD coding, ensuring the solution is both effective and practical for real-world deployment scenarios.

Llama 3.1 [25] belongs to Meta's Llama language model series, designed to enhance performance in natural language understanding and generation. Llama 3.1 distinguishes itself through improved training strategies, larger and more diverse training data, and refined fine-tuning methods, resulting in better accuracy and fluency. Notably, it also supports multimodal inputs and offers enhanced cross-lingual capabilities, making it versatile across different languages and types of data.

Qwen 2.5 [26] is an advanced open-source language model developed by Qwen, designed to excel in efficient natural language processing, comprehension, and generation. It is particularly notable for its strong support of Chinese language tasks, making it a valuable tool for applications in Chinese-speaking regions.

Gemma 2 [27] is a lightweight open model that ranges from 2 billion to 27 billion parameters. It incorporates several novel architectural modifications to the Transformer model, including interleaving local-global attentions and group-query attention, which aim to optimize model performance on tasks requiring both localized and global understanding.

4.2   Model Evaluation Metrics

The performance of each model was evaluated using accuracy metrics for three key ICD categories: ICD-10, ICD-O-M, and ICD-O-H. In addition to the individual accuracies for each category, a weighted score was computed as a linear combination of these accuracies, as shown in the following formula:

$$\text{score} = 0.3 \cdot \text{Accuracy}_{\text{ICD-10}} + 0.5 \cdot \text{Accuracy}_{\text{ICD-O-M}} + 0.2 \cdot \text{Accuracy}_{\text{ICD-O-H}} \quad (1)$$

where the individual accuracies are defined as follows:

$$\text{Accuracy}_{\text{ICD-10}} = \frac{\text{Number of correct ICD-10 codes}}{\text{Total number of samples}} \quad (2)$$

$$\text{Accuracy}_{\text{ICD-O-M}} = \frac{\text{Number of correct ICD-O-M codes}}{\text{Total number of samples}} \quad (3)$$

$$\text{Accuracy}_{\text{ICD-O-H}} = \frac{\text{Number of correct ICD-O-H codes}}{\text{Total number of samples}} \quad (4)$$

Thus, the final evaluation score is a weighted average of the accuracies for ICD-10, ICD-O-M, and ICD-O-H, reflecting their relative importance in the overall model performance.

4.3   Results

Table 2 presents the performance of the baseline models, along with their performance when CoT reasoning is applied. The results indicate that, in complex tasks, prompts optimized for a specific LLM do not generalize well to other LLMs. While CoT reasoning enhances interpretability and accuracy within the targeted model, its effectiveness diminishes when applied to different models. This suggests that CoT prompts need to be tailored to the unique characteristics of each model to achieve optimal performance, especially in categories like ICD-O, which require detailed reasoning and decision-making.

Table 2. Results of ICD Coding Task Across Models.

Model	ICD-10(Acc)	ICD-O-M(Acc)	ICD-O-H(Acc)	score
Llama3.1:8b	0.7593	0.7593	0.7407	0.7556
Llama3.1:8b CoT	0.6852	0.7407	0.7407	0.7241
Qwen2.5:7b	0.7778	0.7778	0.7407	0.7704
Qwen2.5:7b CoT	0.6852	0.6852	0.7407	0.6963
Gemma2:9b	0.7963	0.8333	0.7778	0.8111
Gemma2:9b CoT	0.5556	0.5556	0.7778	0.6
Qwen2.5:14b	0.8519	0.8333	0.8148	0.8352
Qwen2.5:14b CoT	**0.9074**	**0.9074**	**0.8519**	**0.8963**

5   Discussion

The results presented in Table 2 highlight the significant strengths of CoT reasoning in improving interpretability and accuracy for automated ICD coding, particularly when applied to models that have been specifically optimized for it. However, despite these strengths, there are limitations to consider.

5.1   Limitations

Four limitations were identified in our study:

1. **Model-Specific CoT Optimization:** CoT prompts optimized for one model may not yield the same benefits when applied to other models. This variability is due to differences in the internal representations and processing mechanisms across different LLMs.
2. **Need for High Reasoning Capability:** CoT reasoning requires models to perform complex, multi-step logical inferences, which demand advanced reasoning capabilities. Larger models, with their increased parameter counts and enhanced representational capacity, are generally better suited for such tasks.
3. **Handling of Complex Cases:** For complex medical cases, particularly those involving comorbidities or rare diseases, the automated coding system may struggle to fully comprehend and correctly assign ICD codes. Such cases require more nuanced clinical judgment and detailed information, which often fall outside the capabilities of an automated system.
4. **Adaptation to Regional Differences:** ICD coding standards can vary by country or region due to differences in healthcare policies and practices. As a result, automated coding systems may require localization to account for the specific diagnostic standards and practices of different regions or healthcare systems.

5.2   Error Analysis

Error analysis was conducted when performing lymphoma ICD coding. The errors were categorized into three distinct types, as outlined in Table 3. Models are prone to overlooking critical aspects of clinical information, including specific diagnostic details, standard terminologies such as "Not Otherwise Specified (NOS)", and distinguishing between closely related subtypes. These tendencies highlight the challenges in capturing fine-grained distinctions, adhering to standardized ICD coding criteria, and resolving ambiguities in closely overlapping categories.

5.3   Future Work

Four avenues for future work emerge from the findings of this study:

Table 3. Error categories.

Type	Prediction	Answer
Neglect of Disease Details	Follicular Lymphoma	Follicular Lymphoma Grade IIIa
Neglect of Not Other Specified	Diffuse large B-cell lymphoma	Diffuse Non-Hodgkin Lymphoma, NOS
Confusion between Subtypes	Mature T/NK-cell lymphomas, unspecified	Extranodal NK/T-cell lymphoma, nasal type

1. **Generalization of CoT Prompts:** One key direction is to enhance the generalization of CoT prompts across different models. As our results indicate, CoT prompts optimized for one model may not consistently transfer to others. Future research could focus on developing more adaptive or dynamic CoT prompting techniques that are tailored to the specific characteristics of individual models. This could potentially improve the transferability and effectiveness of CoT reasoning across a wider range of LLMs.
2. **Handling Complex Medical Cases:** As automated ICD coding systems may struggle with complex cases, particularly those involving comorbidities or rare diseases, future work could explore the integration of more advanced reasoning capabilities or domain-specific expertise. One approach could involve leveraging hybrid models that combine the strengths of LLMs with traditional rule-based systems or clinical decision support systems to better handle complex medical scenarios.
3. **Adaptation to Regional and Policy Variations:** The adaptability of ICD coding systems to different regional standards and healthcare policies is another important area for future work. Developing localized models that can adjust to the specific diagnostic and coding practices of different countries or regions would enhance the applicability of automated ICD coding systems in diverse healthcare environments.
4. **Continuous Updates and Learning:** The periodic updates to the ICD system, such as changes in disease classifications or new medical standards, highlight the need for continuous model retraining and knowledge base updates. Future work could investigate approaches for enabling LLMs to automatically adapt to changes in coding standards without requiring manual intervention. This could be achieved through techniques like continual learning or incremental knowledge integration.

6   Conclusion

In this study, we developed the application of CoT reasoning in automated ICD coding of lymphoma cases, utilizing a variety of LLMs including Llama 3.1, Qwen 2.5, and Gemma 2. Our results demonstrate that while CoT reasoning can enhance interpretability and accuracy within the specific model it is optimized for, its effectiveness is limited when applied to other models. This limitation suggests that CoT prompts should be customized to each model's unique architecture and capabilities for optimal performance.

Our research contributes to the ongoing exploration of CoT reasoning as a method for enhancing LLM-based ICD coding systems. We provide evidence that model-specific CoT prompt optimization is crucial for achieving reliable performance, and we encourage future work to focus on developing adaptive CoT strategies to enable broader applicability across diverse models. By advancing our understanding of CoT reasoning in LLMs, this study lays the groundwork for further innovations in automated medical coding, ultimately supporting more efficient and accurate healthcare documentation.

Acknowledgments. This study is supported by National Natural Science Foundation of China (62302151) and Fundamental Research Funds for the Central Universities (B220202076).

References

1. Gao, X., He, P., Zhou, Y., Qin, X.: Artificial intelligence applications in smart healthcare: a survey. Future Internet **16**(9), 308 (2024)
2. Harrison, J.E., Weber, S., Jakob, R., Chute, C.G.: ICD-11: an international classification of diseases for the twenty-first century. BMC Med. Inform. Decis. Mak. **21**, 1–10 (2021)
3. Madden, J.M., Lakoma, M.D., Rusinak, D., Lu, C.Y., Soumerai, S.B.: Missing clinical and behavioral health data in a large electronic health record (EHR) system. J. Am. Med. Inform. Assoc. **23**(6), 1143–1149 (2016)
4. Teng, F., Liu, Y., Li, T., Zhang, Y., Li, S., Zhao, Y.: A review on deep neural networks for ICD coding. IEEE Trans. Knowl. Data Eng. **35**(5), 4357–4375 (2022)
5. Kavuluru, R., Rios, A., Lu, Y.: An empirical evaluation of supervised learning approaches in assigning diagnosis codes to electronic medical records. Artif. Intell. Med. **65**(2), 155–166 (2015)
6. Ong, J., et al.: Applying large language model artificial intelligence for retina international classification of diseases (ICD) coding. J. Med. Artif. Intell. **6** (2023)
7. Chen, C., Haupert, S.R., Zimmermann, L., Shi, X., Fritsche, L.G., Mukherjee, B.: Global prevalence of post-coronavirus disease 2019 (COVID-19) condition or long COVID: a meta-analysis and systematic review. J. Infect. Dis. **226**(9), 1593–1607 (2022)
8. Li, J., Lai, S., Gao, G.F., Shi, W.: The emergence, genomic diversity and global spread of SARS-CoV-2. Nature **600**(7889), 408–418 (2021)
9. Wei, J., et al.: Chain-of-thought prompting elicits reasoning in large language models. Adv. Neural. Inf. Process. Syst. **35**, 24824–24837 (2022)
10. Brown, T.B.: Language models are few-shot learners. arXiv preprint arXiv:2005.14165 (2020)
11. Achiam, J., et al.: GPT-4 technical report. arXiv preprint arXiv:2303.08774 (2023)
12. Singhal, K., et al.: Large language models encode clinical knowledge. Nature **620**(7972), 172–180 (2023)
13. Singhal, K., et al.: Towards expert-level medical question answering with large language models. arXiv preprint arXiv:2305.09617 (2023)

14. Jin, D., Pan, E., Oufattole, N., Weng, W.H., Fang, H., Szolovits, P.: What disease does this patient have? A large-scale open domain question answering dataset from medical exams. Appl. Sci. **11**(14), 6421 (2021)
15. Li, Y., Li, Z., Zhang, K., Dan, R., Jiang, S., Zhang, Y.: ChatDoctor: a medical chat model fine-tuned on a large language model meta-AI (LLaMA) using medical domain knowledge. Cureus **15**(6) (2023)
16. Han, T., et al.: MedAlpaca–an open-source collection of medical conversational ai models and training data. arXiv preprint arXiv:2304.08247 (2023)
17. Wu, C., Zhang, X., Zhang, Y., Wang, Y., Xie, W.: PMC-LLaMA: further finetuning llama on medical papers. arXiv preprint arXiv:2304.14454 **2**(5), 6 (2023)
18. Kojima, T., Gu, S.S., Reid, M., Matsuo, Y., Iwasawa, Y.: Large language models are zero-shot reasoners. Adv. Neural. Inf. Process. Syst. **35**, 22199–22213 (2022)
19. Bi, Z., Zhang, N., Jiang, Y., Deng, S., Zheng, G., Chen, H.: When do program-of-thought works for reasoning? In: Proceedings of the AAAI Conference on Artificial Intelligence, vol. 38, pp. 17691–17699 (2024)
20. Cheng, Z., et al.: Binding language models in symbolic languages. arXiv preprint arXiv:2210.02875 (2022)
21. Imani, S., Du, L., Shrivastava, H.: MathPrompter: mathematical reasoning using large language models. arXiv preprint arXiv:2303.05398 (2023)
22. Chen, Z., Zhou, Q., Shen, Y., Hong, Y., Zhang, H., Gan, C.: See, think, confirm: interactive prompting between vision and language models for knowledge-based visual reasoning. arXiv preprint arXiv:2301.05226 (2023)
23. Farkas, R., Szarvas, G.: Automatic construction of rule-based ICD-9-CM coding systems. In: BMC Bioinformatics, vol. 9, pp. 1–9. Springer (2008)
24. Zong, H., et al.: Advancing Chinese biomedical text mining with community challenges. J. Biomed. Inform. 104716 (2024)
25. Dubey, A., et al.: The LLaMA 3 herd of models. arXiv preprint arXiv:2407.21783 (2024)
26. Yang, A., et al.: Qwen2 technical report. arXiv preprint arXiv:2407.10671 (2024)
27. Team, G., et al.: Gemma 2: improving open language models at a practical size. arXiv preprint arXiv:2408.00118 (2024)

Harnessing Retrieval-Augmented LLMs for Training-Free Tumor Coding Classification

Zhenyu Ge and Ning Han$^{(\boxtimes)}$

Xiangtan University, Xiangtan, China
{zhenyuge,ninghan}@xtu.edu.cn

Abstract. Tumor coding classification (TCC) aims to systematically classify and code tumor diseases based on their characteristics, facilitating the statistical analysis and communication of medical information. Existing research typically relies on training deep models to learn normal distributions, whether in supervised or unsupervised settings. However, these training-based methods are often domain-specific, leading to high deployment costs, as any changes in the domain require new data collection and model retraining. In this paper, we radically depart from previous approaches and propose a tumor coding classification method based on large language models (LLMs), introducing a novel, training-free paradigm called TCC-LLMs. This method integrates a re-trainedretrieval-augmented generation pipeline with LLMs to enhance the accuracy of malignant tumor coding classification tasks. Specifically, we first use pre-trained LLMs to extract key pathological staging features from patient records. Then, based on these features and a pre-trained vector database, we retrieve tumor codes that match the pathological stages. Finally, we leverage LLMs to reorder the retrieved tumor codes and determine the final code. Our method achieved an accuracy of 89.26% in the 2024 China Health Information Processing Conference evaluation task, securing fourth place. Our code is available at https://github.com/MagicCat-AI/Chip2024-Tumor-Coding-Classification.

Keywords: Large Language Models · Retrieval-Augmented Generation · Tumor Coding Classification

1 Introduction

The Tumor Coding Classification (TCC) task aims to systematically classify and code tumors based on their characteristics. It is essential for organizing and categorizing cancer-related diseases according to standardized coding systems, thereby enabling accurate data analysis, efficient communication, and informed decision-making in medical practice and research. As highlighted in a study reviewing the latest advancements in the Chinese Biomedical Text Mining Community Challenge [27], this underscores the importance of the TCC task and

© The Author(s), under exclusive license to Springer Nature Singapore Pte Ltd. 2025
Y. Zhang et al. (Eds.): CHIP 2024, CCIS 2458, pp. 117–129, 2025.
https://doi.org/10.1007/978-981-96-4298-4_11

its role in enhancing the efficiency of medical data processing. Recently, Large language models (LLMs) have achieved significant success in both academia and industry, with widespread applications in tasks such as text classification, machine translation, and question answering. Their powerful capabilities in natural language understanding and generation have made them indispensable tools. Recently, advancements in large-scale models, such as ChatGLM by Zhipu AI [6] and Qwen by Baidu Wenxin [3], have demonstrated excellent performance, especially in the Chinese language application domain. Nonetheless, the scarcity and high ambiguity of tumor coding data make it challenging for fine-tuned large models to meet the demands of real-world applications.

LLM-based methods still encounter considerable challenges when applied to specialized tasks like tumor coding classification. In text classification tasks, most existing research focuses on fine-tuning large language models or leveraging prompt engineering. In the case of tumor coding classification, Iannantuono et al. [8] note that even advanced LLMs capabilities may not fully capture the nuances of the task or the specific instructions required. Medical data, particularly tumor coding, has unique characteristics that make the direct application of retrieval-based methods more complex. Medical records are often highly structured and domain-specific, frequently containing terminology or jargon that general retrieval systems may struggle to match. Moreover, the coding process itself demands a deep understanding of medical knowledge and detailed rules of coding systems such as ICD-10. As such, a key challenge is the lack of high-quality, up-to-date tumor coding datasets for model fine-tuning. Furthermore, the high ambiguity between codes further complicates the task. While Retrieval-Augmented Generation (RAG) methods, as shown by Lewis et al. [13], hold promise in addressing similar challenges in other domains, training-based methods are typically domain-specific, resulting in high deployment costs, as any change in domain requires new data collection and model retraining. These considerations led us to explore a novel research question: *Can we develop a training-free TCC method?*

In this paper, we aim to address this challenging problem. Developing a training-free TCC model is difficult due to the lack of clear domain-specific priors for the target setting. However, such priors can be captured using large foundational models, which are known for their generalization capabilities and vast knowledge encodings. Therefore, we explored the potential of combining the existing RAG process with LLMs to solve the training-free TCC problem. Based on our preliminary findings, we propose the first training-free language-based TCC method, called TCC-LLMs, which jointly leverages pretrained RAG and LLMs for TCC. Specifically, we first use pretrained LLMs to extract key pathological staging features from patient records. Then, based on these features and a pretrained vector database, we retrieve tumor codes that match the pathological stages. Finally, we use LLMs to re-rank the retrieved tumor codes and determine the final code. Our method achieved an accuracy of 89.26% in the 2024 China Health Information Processing Conference evaluation task, ranking fourth.

Our contributions are thus two-fold: 1) We investigate, for the first time, the problem of training-free tumor coding classification, advocating its importance for the deployment of tumor coding classification systems in real settings where data collection may not be possible. 2) We propose an innovative approach that integrates the RAG pipeline with LLMs, specifically designed for Training-free tumor coding classification. Extensive experiments conduct on a standard benchmark to validate the effectiveness of TCC-LLMs.

2   Related Work

2.1   Text Classification

Medical text classification, as one of the important applications in the field of Natural Language Processing (NLP), has garnered increasing attention from researchers. By deeply analyzing medical text datasets, researchers have sought to apply these techniques to disease classification, clinical diagnosis, patient record analysis, and other areas.In the early stages of research, medical text classification primarily relied on traditional machine learning methods [16,22,25], such as Support Vector Machines (SVM), Naive Bayes classifiers, Decision Trees, and K-Nearest Neighbors (KNN). For instance, Wang et al. [22] typically utilized handcrafted features like TF-IDF (Term Frequency-Inverse Document Frequency) and the Bag-of-Words (BoW) model for text representation. However, the effectiveness of these traditional methods was constrained by the quality of the text features. This limitation was especially pronounced when addressing the complex terminology and diverse text structures in the medical domain, making it difficult to fully capture the deep semantic information within the text. In recent years, with the advancement of deep learning technologies, medical text classification has made significant progress. Convolutional Neural Networks (CNN), Recurrent Neural Networks (RNN), Long Short-Term Memory networks (LSTM), Bidirectional Encoder Representation of Transformer, and LLMs have been widely applied in text analysis [7,12,17,25]. Compared to traditional methods, deep learning models are capable of automatically extracting higher-level features from the text through an end-to-end learning process, thus significantly improving classification performance. These methods have driven the development of medical text classification.

2.2   Large Language Models (LLMs)

With the advent of the Transformer architecture [20], large language models containing hundreds of billions of parameters, trained on massive text datasets, have achieved remarkable performance across a wide range of tasks. Notable examples include GPT-4 [1], PaLM2 [2], and LLaMA [19]. These models demonstrate strong capabilities in understanding natural language and solving complex tasks through text generation, including in the medical field. Thirunavukarasu et al. [18] discuss how large language models can be used in clinical settings, considering both their advantages and limitations, as well as their potential to improve the efficiency and effectiveness of medical clinical practice, education, and research.

However, due to the need for specialized medical knowledge in the healthcare domain, LLMs have not yet fully realized their potential in biomedical tasks. To address this issue, various methods are proposed. Wang et al. [21] use generated QA (question-answering) instances for supervised fine-tuning to help large language models learn the specialized knowledge of traditional Chinese medicine. Ye et al. [24] apply RAG to further enhance the performance of the fine-tuned models. These methods make significant contributions to the development of medical-application LLMs.

2.3 Retrieval-Augmented Generation (RAG)

Retrieval-Augmented Generation (RAG) is an advanced framework that combines the strengths of retrieval-based and generative models to enhance performance on tasks that require rich knowledge and contextual understanding [5,13]. The concept was first introduced to address the limitations of traditional generative models, which rely solely on their pre-trained knowledge, making it challenging for them to produce accurate or domain-specific outputs in knowledge-intensive tasks. RAG operates by retrieving relevant external documents or pieces of information from a knowledge base, such as a vector database, and then using a generative model to synthesize the retrieved information into a coherent response. This approach enables the model to leverage both vast pre-trained knowledge and external context, improving accuracy, relevance, and interpretability, especially in tasks like question answering, document summarization, and knowledge-intensive natural language processing (NLP) tasks. For instance, Lewis et al. [13] explain that RAG is a technique that helps LLMs generate answers by retrieving information from data sources. RAG combines search techniques with the prompt-based functionality of LLMs, where a question is posed to the model, and information found through a search algorithm is used as contextual background. This query and the contextual information retrieved are integrated into the prompt sent to LLMs. This approach effectively addresses specific tasks, particularly in the case of tumor coding and classification tasks, as discussed in the paper. Jeong et al. [9] mention that when applying existing large model methods to medical-specific tasks, poor generalization becomes evident, leading to the retrieval of incorrect documents or making inaccurate judgments. Therefore, they propose a medical-specific RAG framework. Ye et al. [24] utilize the RAG technique to improve the model's ability to perform medical tasks.

3 Method

3.1 TCC-LLMs

Given the complexity of lymphatic task code classification, we have designed a method called TCC-LLMs for tumor coding classification. The premise of this method is the organization and refinement of a knowledge base. This method operates through three main steps: first, extracting the pathology stage from the medical case; second, applying retrieval augmentation based on the extracted pathology stage to gather relevant information; and finally, generating the matched code based on the retrieval results. During this process, the large language model dynamically selects appropriate prompting strategies based on different coding standards, such as ICD-10, ICD-O-M, and ICD-O-H, to ensure accurate generation of results according to the specific coding system.

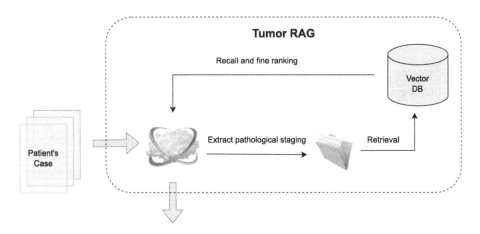

Fig. 1. The overall framework of our TCC-LLMs. It process flow first extracts the pathological staging from the cases, then retrieves the corresponding tumor codes from the vector database, and finally uses the LLMs for r-ranking to obtain the final tumor codes.

Figure 1 shows the specific steps of the TCC-LLMs method. First, patient information is extracted into text input, which is then processed by LLMs for extraction. The resulting pathology stage is passed to the embedding model, which matches the corresponding codes in Faiss. The matched codes from Faiss are then passed back to the embedding model, which provides the possible codes for evaluation by LLMs. Finally, the LLMs outputs the most likely code.

3.2 Basic LLMs

Participants in the competition are allowed to use all available open-source large language models. This selection process is not arbitrary but is based on a thorough evaluation of each model's performance in various tasks. Considering the capability to process Chinese medical cases, we ultimately select two outstanding representatives from domestic open-source large models: ChatGLM-Plus from Zhipu AI [6] and Qwen-Max from Tongyi Qianwen [3]. Both models are based on the powerful Transformer architecture, which was inspired by the design principles of [20], a model that revolutionized traditional sequential models in the field of natural language processing. After a comprehensive comparison of ChatGLM-Plus and Qwen-Max in terms of language understanding, generation quality, response speed, and adaptability to complex contexts, we select these two models. Based on the architecture of the Transformer, they are continuously optimized and trained, achieving excellent performance in specific tasks, and providing reliable technical support for our work.

3.3   Prompt Format

A prompt is a natural language sequence used to assist LLMs in generating responses and completing a specified task. Studies [11,23] show that well-crafted prompts are of significant importance for the performance of LLMs on specific tasks, as the construction of the prompt has a major impact on the model's output. Moreover, to handle tasks in specific domains, a formatted large model prompt is often required, consisting of a task description and several task examples as demonstrations. For retrieval-augmented generation-based large language models, the prompts typically include the correct answers. In their work, Liu et al. [14] study such prompts and how to construct relevant ones. Mesko et al. [15], in their research, focus on prompts for medical-oriented large language models. Building on their work, in our approach, we apply prompt engineering to two distinct environments: one for extracting pathological staging from patient cases, and another for analyzing and matching pathological staging with possible coding retrieved from external sources. Below are examples of these prompts.

```
prompt = '''
任务目标：查看病人的病例并分析病人肿瘤的病例诊断
任务要求：
    1、要求输出尽可能具体的病理诊断和病理分期
    2、病人的病理诊断应该为肿瘤类或者白血病类，如果出现其他类请再次分析病例
    3、如果没有具体的细胞类型，请提供具体的细胞类型

病人的病例：
{}
'''
```

Fig. 2. Prompt templates used by LLMs to extract staging features from patient cases.

As shown in Fig. 2, through continuous experimentation, our prompts can accurately extract the patient's specific pathological stage from the medical case, with almost no hallucination issues.

```
prompt = '''
任务目标: 根据病人的病理{}并根据检索出的{}文档分析病人的{}
任务要求:
    1、先分析病人的病理分期再结合文档回答问题
    2、病人的{}只存在一个
    3、若检索出的文档不包含用户问题的答案，你必须选择一个检索结果
    4、要求更加具体地选择而不是更加广泛地选择
检索出的文档:
{}
'''
```

Fig. 3. Prompt templates used by LLMs to analyze tumor codes and generate final coding.

As shown in Fig. 3, our prompts help the large model to match the pathological stage and coding, given the pathological stage of the known patient and the retrieval results.

3.4   Retrieval-Augmented Generation

In the studies by [4] and [26], the current advancements and limitations of RAG technology are discussed. Based on their findings and considering the characteristic of a small dataset, we opt for traditional RAG methods. Although [10] provides an approach using long-context RAG, we find that this method results in poor generalization on the test set due to its inability to correctly extract the pathological staging. Therefore, we choose to first use a large model to extract the pathological staging from the cases, and then apply RAG for the pathological staging generation.

The RAG method consists of three steps: retrieval, augmentation, and generation.

Retrieval: In this step, relevant context is retrieved from external knowledge sources based on the user's query. To achieve this, we use an embedding model to embed the user's query into the same vector space as other context in the vector database, as shown in Fig. 4. This allows for similarity search and returns the top-k most similar data objects from the vector database.

Augmentation: The user's query and the retrieved additional context are then filled into a prompt template.

Generation: Finally, the retrieval-augmented prompt is input into the large language model for generation. In our tumor coding classification task, we use Faiss as our vector database and gte-large-zh as our embedding model for retrieval. We embed known tumor codes and their corresponding cases into the vector database. The embedding model then matches the cases provided by the large language model to the tumor codes in the vector database. Lastly, the potential tumor codes are returned to the large language model for analysis.

C80.0   恶性肿瘤，原发部位不明

C80.9   （全身性）癌（症/病）（原发/继发）多

C80.9   发性癌症NOS部位（原发/继发）

C80.9   恶性恶病质/原发部位NOS（未写明原发部位不明）

C81.0   结节性淋巴细胞为主型[NLPHL]

C81.1   结节硬化型（经典型）[NSHL]

C81.2   混合细胞型（经典型）[MCHL]

C81.3   淋巴细胞减少/消减型（经典型）[LDHL]

C81.4   富于淋巴细胞型（经典型）[LRCHL]，除外：结节性淋巴细胞为主型

C81.7   （经典型）霍奇金淋巴瘤[CHL]，其他型

C81.9   霍奇金淋巴瘤NOS

C82.0   滤泡性淋巴瘤I级/小分裂细胞，滤泡性

Fig. 4. A portion of the ICD-10 coding knowledge base.

4   Experiment

4.1   Experimental Settings

Datasets. We conduct tumor coding classification experiments on CHIP 2024 Lymphoma Information Extraction. The dataset consists of 54 training samples and 108 test samples, with each sample as shown in Fig. 5. Each sample contains three key metrics: ICD-10, ICD-O-H, and ICD-O-M. We establish a knowledge base related to the dataset. We extract the pathological staging of the case, pass the pathological stage to the embedding model for retrieval in Faiss, and then the large language model performs the final analysis to confirm the coding classification. We evaluate the accuracy of ChatGLM-Plus and Qwen-Max on this task.

Evaluation Metrics. We adopt the widely used Accuracy as the evaluation metric. The Accuracy of each part of the tumor code is calculated separately, and the overall Accuracy is computed according to the corresponding coefficients. The specific calculation formula is as

$$\text{Acc}_{\text{total}} = w_1 \cdot \text{Acc}_{\text{ICD-10}} + w_2 \cdot \text{Acc}_{\text{ICD-O-H}} + w_3 \cdot \text{Acc}_{\text{ICD-O-M}}. \tag{1}$$

The formula above represents the task's accuracy score as the weighted sum of the classification accuracy scores for each category, where (w1) is 0.3, (w2) is 0.2, and (w3) is 0.5. The accuracy for each category is calculated using as

$$\text{Acc} = \frac{\text{Number of Correctly Classified Samples}}{\text{Total Number of Samples}} \times 100\%. \tag{2}$$

We can obtain the Acc metric for the task through the calculation of these two formulas, which serves as a criterion for evaluating the model's and method's performance in the tumor coding classification task.

"id":"s001",

"text":   ""噬血细胞综合征(hemophagocytic syndrome，HPS)又称噬血细胞性淋巴组织细胞增多症

　　　一、一般资料

患者，女性，60岁，因"头晕乏力1个月余，发热1d"入院。患者1个月前......

二、检查。

2023年3月8日血常规:血红蛋白54 g/L;血小板计数77x109/L...

三、诊断与鉴别诊断

根据上述结果最终诊断:1.弥漫大B细胞淋巴瘤IV期(AnnArbor 4B期IPI 4分....·

四、治疗

患者初诊考虑为Evans综合征，激素治疗有效，随访中出现血小板及血红蛋白......

五、治疗结果、随访及转归

患者经R-CHOP方案4个疗程评估后达到CR，目前化疗......"",

"date of first diagnosis":"2023年6月15日",

'gender":"女",

"location":"骨髓",

"pathological classification":"弥漫大B细胞性非霍奇金淋巴瘤累及骨髓IV期",

"ICD-10":"C83.3",

"ICD-0-P":"C42.1",

"ICD-0-M":"9680/3",

"ICD-O-H":"6"

Fig. 5. This is a data entry from our dataset, and we need to extract its text features.

Implementation Details. Our TCC-LLMs method leverages the pre-trained Qwen-MAX[1] as the large language model within the retrieval-augmented generation framework, Faiss[2] as the vector database, and the pre-trained gte-large-zh[3] as the embedding model. In this approach, we utilize the Faiss vector database, which is based on efficient data compression and quantization techniques, to store and retrieve tumor codes. The retrieved codes are then re-ranked by Qwen-MAX to determine the final tumor code.

Table 1. Comparison of top 10 methods accuracy.

Model	ICD-10	ICD-O-H	ICD-O-M
TOP-1	0.9259	0.9444	0.9259
TOP-2	0.8889	0.9630	0.9259
TOP-3	0.9074	0.8519	0.9074
TOP-4 (TCC-LLMs)	**0.8704**	**0.8889**	**0.9074**
TOP-5	0.8519	0.8519	0.8889
TOP-6	0.8889	0.7963	0.8704
TOP-7	0.7778	0.9074	0.8889
TOP-8	0.8148	0.8519	0.8704
TOP-9	0.7778	0.7593	0.8519
TOP-10	0.6667	0.8333	0.7593

4.2 Performance Comparison

In Table 1, we compare the classification accuracy results of the top 10 methods from the 2024 China Health Information Processing Conference evaluation task. The results show that our method ranked 4th, highlighting its strong competitiveness among all approaches.

4.3 Ablation Study

We conducted an ablation study on the different large models used in our approach. As shown in Table 2, the Qwen-Max model consistently outperforms the ChatGLM-Plus model in the tumor coding classification task, demonstrating superior accuracy across all coding categories. These results validate the effectiveness of the Qwen-Max model for tumor coding classification. Furthermore, we compared the performance of Qwen-Max based on RAG (i.e., our TCC-LLMs) with that of using the Qwen-Max model directly for case analysis. As

---

[1] https://tongyi.aliyun.com/qianwen/.

[2] https://ai.meta.com/tools/faiss/.

[3] https://huggingface.co/thenlper/gte-large-zh.

shown in the table, the methods of ChatGLM-Plus + TCC-LLMs and Qwen-Max + TCC-LLMs outperformed the direct use of ChatGLM-Plus and Qwen-Max across all three coding categories. This confirms the effectiveness of our TCC-LLMs method, which integrates the Retrieval-Augmented Generation pipeline with Large Language Models.

Table 2. Comparison of different LLMs and integrated RAG.

Model	ICD-10	ICD-O-H	ICD-O-M
ChatGLM-Plus	0.203	0.148	0.074
Qwen-Max	0.351	0.296	0.203
ChatGLM-Plus + TCC-LLMs	0.759	0.796	0.722
Qwen-Max + TCC-LLMs	0.87	0.889	0.907

4.4   Limitations

To further strengthen our manuscript, we have conducted an analysis of failure cases where tumor coding errors occurred due to hallucinations, incorrect retrievals, or improper coding decisions. For instance, when using the prompt in Fig. 2 for case 5, involving diffuse large B-cell non-Hodgkin lymphoma with bone marrow involvement at stage IV, the model occasionally exhibits hallucinations, leading to the pathological stage being misidentified as another type of non-Hodgkin lymphoma. In other cases, even when the model correctly identifies the pathological stage, erroneous retrieval from the knowledge base may return codes that omit the correct one. These challenges underscore key limitations within our RAG-enhanced tumor coding classification system.

Hallucinations: In some instances, the model generated information that was not grounded in the provided context or knowledge base. This phenomenon, known as hallucination, can lead to incorrect coding decisions. Detailed examination of these cases revealed that they often occurred when the input query was ambiguous or contained insufficient information. To mitigate this issue, future work could focus on improving the robustness of the retrieval mechanism and enhancing the quality control checks on generated outputs.

Erroneous Retrievals: Errors in the retrieval process can result in the model accessing irrelevant or outdated information from the knowledge base. We found that such errors were more common with less frequent or rare tumor types. Addressing this limitation might involve refining the search algorithms used by the RAG model or expanding the knowledge base with more comprehensive data on rare tumors.

Incorrect Coding Choices: Despite the advanced capabilities of our RAG-based approach, there were instances where the model selected incorrect codes for tumor classification. These failures were often linked to ambiguities in the medical terminology or variations in how different institutions code similar conditions. Future improvements could include incorporating feedback mechanisms from domain experts to refine the decision-making process and reduce the incidence of such errors.

5   Conclusion

This paper explores the evaluation of a training-free tumor coding classification task based on pre-trained Retrieval-Augmented Generation models and introduces a method called TCC-LLMs. This method requires the organization and refinement of the knowledge base. Specifically, we use pre-trained LLMs to extract key pathological staging features from patient records. Based on a pre-trained vector database and leveraging the reasoning capabilities of LLMs, we re-rank the retrieved tumor codes to determine the final tumor code. In the 2024 China Health Information Processing Conference evaluation task, our method achieved an excellent ranking, validating its effectiveness. In the future, we plan to further explore the explainability of agent-based systems in the medical field and their potential for intelligent applications.

Acknowledgments. This work is supported by the National Natural Science Foundation of China (No. 62272156), and the Natural Science Foundation of Hunan Province (No. 2024JJ6435).

References

1. Achiam, J., et al.: GPT-4 technical report. arXiv preprint arXiv:2303.08774 (2023)
2. Anil, R., et al.: Palm 2 technical report. arXiv preprint arXiv:2305.10403 (2023)
3. Bai, J., et al.: Qwen technical report. arXiv preprint arXiv:2309.16609 (2023)
4. Cai, D., Wang, Y., Liu, L., Shi, S.: Recent advances in retrieval-augmented text generation. In: Proceedings of the 45th International ACM SIGIR Conference on Research and Development in Information Retrieval, pp. 3417–3419 (2022)
5. Gao, Y., et al.: Retrieval-augmented generation for large language models: a survey. arXiv preprint arXiv:2312.10997 (2023)
6. GLM, T., et al.: ChatGLM: a family of large language models from GLM-130B to GLM-4 all tools. arXiv preprint arXiv:2406.12793 (2024)
7. Han, N., Chen, J., Xiao, G., Zhang, H., Zeng, Y., Chen, H.: Fine-grained cross-modal alignment network for text-video retrieval. In: Proceedings of the 29th ACM International Conference on Multimedia, pp. 3826–3834 (2021)
8. Iannantuono, G.M., Bracken-Clarke, D., Floudas, C.S., Roselli, M., Gulley, J.L., Karzai, F.: Applications of large language models in cancer care: current evidence and future perspectives. Front. Oncol. **13**, 1268915 (2023)
9. Jeong, M., Sohn, J., Sung, M., Kang, J.: Improving medical reasoning through retrieval and self-reflection with retrieval-augmented large language models. Bioinformatics **40**(Supplement_1), i119–i129 (2024)

10. Jiang, Z., Ma, X., Chen, W.: LongRAG: enhancing retrieval-augmented generation with long-context LLMs. arXiv preprint arXiv:2406.15319 (2024)
11. Jin, W., Cheng, Y., Shen, Y., Chen, W., Ren, X.: A good prompt is worth millions of parameters: low-resource prompt-based learning for vision-language models. arXiv preprint arXiv:2110.08484 (2021)
12. Johnson, R., Zhang, T.: Deep pyramid convolutional neural networks for text categorization. In: Proceedings of the 55th Annual Meeting of the Association for Computational Linguistics (Volume 1: Long Papers), pp. 562–570 (2017)
13. Lewis, P., et al.: Retrieval-augmented generation for knowledge-intensive NLP tasks. Adv. Neural. Inf. Process. Syst. **33**, 9459–9474 (2020)
14. Liu, P., Yuan, W., Fu, J., Jiang, Z., Hayashi, H., Neubig, G.: Pre-train, prompt, and predict: a systematic survey of prompting methods in natural language processing. ACM Comput. Surv. **55**(9), 1–35 (2023)
15. Meskó, B.: Prompt engineering as an important emerging skill for medical professionals: tutorial. J. Med. Internet Res. **25**, e50638 (2023)
16. Rubinstein, B.I., Bartlett, P.L., Huang, L., Taft, N.: Learning in a large function space: Privacy-preserving mechanisms for SVM learning. J. Priv. Confidentiality **4**(1) (2012)
17. Song, Y., Zhang, J., Tian, Z., Yang, Y., Huang, M., Li, D.: LLM-based privacy data augmentation guided by knowledge distillation with a distribution tutor for medical text classification. arXiv preprint arXiv:2402.16515 (2024)
18. Thirunavukarasu, A.J., Ting, D., Elangovan, K., Gutierrez, L., Tan, T.F., Ting, D.: Large language models in medicine. Nat. Med. **29**(8), 1930–1940 (2023)
19. Touvron, H., et al.: LLaMA: open and efficient foundation language models. arXiv preprint arXiv:2302.13971 (2023)
20. Vaswani, A.: Attention is all you need. Adv. Neural Inf. Process. Syst. (2017)
21. Wang, H., et al.: Huatuo: tuning LLaMA model with Chinese medical knowledge. arXiv preprint arXiv:2304.06975 (2023)
22. Wang, S., Hou, Y., Li, Z., Dong, J., Tang, C.: Combining convnets with handcrafted features for action recognition based on an HMM-SVM classifier. Multimed. Tools Appl. **77**, 18983–18998 (2018)
23. White, J., et al.: A prompt pattern catalog to enhance prompt engineering with chatGPT. arXiv preprint arXiv:2302.11382 (2023)
24. Ye, Q., et al.: Qilin-med: multi-stage knowledge injection advanced medical large language model. arXiv preprint arXiv:2310.09089 (2023)
25. Zhang, S., Zheng, D., Hu, X., Yang, M.: Bidirectional long short-term memory networks for relation classification. In: Proceedings of the 29th Pacific Asia Conference on Language, Information and Computation, pp. 73–78 (2015)
26. Zhao, P., et al.: Retrieval-augmented generation for AI-generated content: a survey. arXiv preprint arXiv:2402.19473 (2024)
27. Zong, H., et al.: Advancing Chinese biomedical text mining with community challenges. J. Biomed. Inform. 104716 (2024)

Hierarchical Information Extraction and Classification of Lymphoma Tumor Codes Based On LLM

Wenjie Fang[1], Chengyan Wu[2], Yufei Cheng[3], and Ying Li[4(✉)]

[1] Nanhai Maternity and Children's Hospital Affiliated to Guangzhou, University of Traditional Chinese Medicine, Foshan, China
[2] School of Electronic Science and Engineering, South China Normal University, Foshan, China
[3] School of Business, Yangzhou University, Yangzhou, China
[4] GuangDong Women and Children Hospital, Guangzhou, China
liyinggdsfy@163.com

Abstract. The medical information extraction task plays a crucial role in assisting doctors by extracting patient-related information from clinical cases. Detailed processing of the extracted data enables the identification of key information within medical records. Through comprehensive analysis, the model can determine the specific disease affecting the patient, thereby providing valuable reference information to clinicians and alleviating their workload. In this paper, we present a medical information extraction and classification framework developed for an open competition task at the 10th Conference on Health Information Processing (CHIP 2024). This task involves processing complex and information-dense patient case texts to extract the specific lymphoma diagnosis and subsequently generate tumor codes based on the extracted lymphoma information and other case details. We propose a large model-based framework for information extraction and classification. To tailor the model to this medical task, we fine-tune it using an augmented dataset. To facilitate accurate extraction of information relevant to code generation, we employ a chain-of-thought (CoT) approach, guiding the model to incrementally extract key information. Given the inherent challenges in generative tasks, such as the risk of producing similar but incorrect codes, we transform the generative task into a classification task. Specifically, the model is tasked with selecting the correct code from a set of possible options, thus improving accuracy. Furthermore, we carefully design and optimize prompt strategies to guide the model in producing reliable outputs. Our experimental results demonstrate that these methodologies enable the model to achieve strong performance in this task.

Keywords: medical information extraction · medical text classification · large language models · data augmentation · chain of thought · instruction fine-tuning

© The Author(s), under exclusive license to Springer Nature Singapore Pte Ltd. 2025
Y. Zhang et al. (Eds.): CHIP 2024, CCIS 2458, pp. 130–145, 2025.
https://doi.org/10.1007/978-981-96-4298-4_12

1   Introduction

With the advancement of automated medical services, the automated processing of medical texts, extraction of medical information, and automatic generation or categorization of patient diseases have rapidly evolved. These advancements aim to build more comprehensive medical records and enhance the convenience of medical consultations for patients. Medical information extraction serves as a foundational task in medical text processing. Traditional methods largely rely on rule-based approaches, which, while effective for specific disease types, often fail to generalize across diverse medical conditions. In recent years, the rise of deep learning has introduced feature-based extraction methods, offering improved generalizability and superior performance across various tasks, provided sufficient training data is available. Once disease-related information is extracted, models can leverage this data to classify the patient's condition. With the increasing prominence of large models in recent years, researchers have explored their applications in medical information extraction and disease classification. Large Language Models (LLMs) have garnered significant attention for their exceptional capabilities in understanding and generating natural language. Unlike smaller language models, LLMs are trained on vast amounts of textual data, enabling them to generalize effectively across a wide range of tasks, including those that are novel or complex. The application of LLMs in clinical diagnosis and medical research represents a cutting-edge and promising frontier. These models hold the potential to improve the efficiency and quality of diagnosis, treatment, and prevention, while also aiding researchers in uncovering new medical insights and methodologies. Notably, LLMs often incorporate extensive foundational medical knowledge, allowing them to process medical information directly. Moreover, by fine-tuning these models on task-specific datasets, they can quickly adapt to specialized applications. Given the high stakes in the medical domain, where errors can have serious consequences, ensuring accuracy and reliability is paramount. The field's stringent compliance requirements further emphasize the need for robust and dependable AI solutions.

The China Health Information Processing Conference (CHIP) brings together researchers and practitioners from academia, industry, and government agencies worldwide to share cutting-edge research, innovative ideas, and successful case studies in the interdisciplinary fields of medical informatics, health informatics, and bioinformatics. CHIP 2024 will continue its tradition of organizing evaluation competitions under the theme of Healthcare Pendant Domain Large Models, providing a platform for researchers to test and showcase their technologies, algorithms, and systems. Task 2 focuses on lymphoma information extraction and tumor registry code generation [1]. Lymphoma, a malignancy originating in the lymphatic system, encompasses a wide range of subtypes and has a high global incidence. Clinical diagnostic coding involves converting diagnostic information into standardized codes, enabling systematic processing and analysis of medical data. This task requires physicians to comprehensively evaluate various clinical details. However, coding lymphoma diagnoses presents significant challenges due to the numerous subtypes, complex characteristics, and varied diagnostic criteria. Large medical models have the potential to assist in clinical diagnostic coding by leveraging extensive medical data to automate the parsing and interpretation of clinical information. These models can provide coding recommendations by simulating the diagnostic reasoning process, offering personalized suggestions that support medical coders. This task aims to evaluate the accuracy and efficiency of large medical models in lymphoma coding. By comparing model-generated codes with those produced by human coders, the study seeks to assess the models' strengths and limitations, thereby advancing their application in clinical practice. Additionally, the growing capabilities of general-purpose large models enable effective extraction of patient pathology information, which can be further utilized for accurate lymphoma code generation.

In Task 2, Lymphoma Information Extraction and Automatic Tumor Coding Generation, we addressed two main challenges: extracting key information from redundant and complex patient cases, and generating accurate tumor codes based on the extracted information. The task was divided into two parts: (1) information extraction from patient cases, and (2) tumor code generation. To tackle these challenges, we employed Qwen2.5-14B-Instruct [2] as our base model. To optimize the model's performance, we first refined the dataset to align with the input format required by large models. Our information extraction process was designed in a two-step chain-of-thought (CoT) approach. In the first step, we extracted lymphoma-related diagnoses and their characteristics from patient cases to form a pathology diagnosis report. In the second step, we used this diagnosis report to extract lymphoma-related diseases and their corresponding categories, effectively breaking down the complex case data into structured and relevant information. This stepwise approach allowed us to focus on extracting specific, useful data before relying on it for further lymphoma-related disease extraction. For the tumor code generation task, we began by augmenting the training data and fine-tuning our model using LoRA to better adapt it to the task. To improve the accuracy of tumor code generation, we converted the generative task into a classification task. Specifically, we adopted a two-stage process: Initial Classification: Based on the previously extracted pathology diagnosis report and lymphoma-related diseases, the model generated the two most likely tumor code categories. These were drawn from a set of all possible tumor coding categories provided as candidate options. Subcategory Classification: For each of the major tumor coding categories, the model selected the most appropriate subcategory. Using the pathology diagnosis report and lymphoma-related disease information as input hints, the model generated the final ICD-10 codes. These were then mapped to their corresponding ICD-O-M codes. For ICD-O-H codes, we directly used the pathology diagnosis report and lymphoma-related diseases as input hints. The model selected the final codes from a predefined list of ICD-O-H options, ensuring accurate classification. This multi-step framework enabled the model to systematically handle complex case data and produce high-quality tumor codes, demonstrating the potential of large models in clinical diagnostic coding tasks.

The main contributions of this work are as follows:

- We utilized Qwen2.5-14B-Instruct as the base model for supervised instruction fine-tuning, leveraging the LoRA framework to enhance model performance. To tailor the model to our specific task, we fine-tuned it using both the training dataset and data augmentation techniques, thereby improving its inference capabilities.
- For patient information extraction, we employed a chain-of-thought (CoT) approach, enabling the model to first retrieve and extract the patient's pathology diagnosis report at a coarse level, before proceeding to the extraction of lymphoma-related diseases and their corresponding categories.
- In the task of automatic tumor code generation, we applied a chain-of-thought methodology to transform the generative task into a classification problem. Initially, the model classified the patient's ICD-10 major categories based on the extracted pathology diagnosis report and lymphoma-related disease information. Subsequently, the model classified the patient into one of the subcategories within the top two major ICD-10 categories.

2 Related Work

2.1 LLMs for Medication

In recent years, large-scale language models (LLMs) have achieved remarkable progress in artificial intelligence. Models such as GPT-3 [3], LLaMA [4], and PaLM [5] have demonstrated exceptional capabilities across various natural language tasks. Despite their impressive performance, key details about their training strategies and parameter configurations remain undisclosed. Although LLaMA is open source, its performance on Chinese tasks is suboptimal due to its predominantly English training corpus.

To address the challenges of applying LLMs to Chinese-specific tasks, Du et al. [6] introduced GLM, an autoregressive pretraining model with 130 billion parameters and multiple training objectives. Building on this, Zeng et al. [7] developed ChatGLM-6B, a bilingual (Chinese-English) dialogue model with 6.2 billion parameters, which is also open source. This study employs ChatGLM2-6B, an enhanced version of ChatGLM-6B, featuring improved performance, extended context handling, and more efficient inference.

Although Large Language Models (LLMs) perform well in general domains, their performance in specialized fields, such as biomedical applications, is often limited due to a lack of domain-specific knowledge. To address this issue, several medical-domain LLMs have been developed.

MedPaLM [8], a variant of PaLM [5], leverages instruction-tuning techniques to provide high-quality answers to medical questions. ChatDoctor [9] fine-tunes LLaMA [4] using both general-purpose datasets and doctor-patient dialogue data to better understand patient needs and offer tailored recommendations. DoctorGLM [10] is a Chinese medical LLM trained on a translated version of ChatDoctor's dataset, employing LoRA [11] to reduce inference time. Similarly,

BenTsao [12], based on LLaMA, fine-tunes its model using both structured and unstructured medical knowledge to ensure factual accuracy in medical QA tasks.

These advancements demonstrate the potential of LLMs to excel in the medical domain by incorporating domain-specific data and fine-tuning techniques.

2.2 Question Answering Task in Medication

In the field of medical natural language processing (NLP), medical information extraction and medical text classification play crucial roles in transforming unstructured clinical data into structured formats for downstream applications. Medical information extraction involves identifying and extracting key entities, such as symptoms, diagnoses, medications, and procedures, from clinical narratives. Numerous studies have addressed this challenge. For instance, An et al. [13] proposed a neural sequence labeling model leveraging Bidirectional LSTM-CRF for clinical entity recognition. Similarly, Singhal et al. [14] introduced a rule-based hybrid model for extracting disease and treatment relations from clinical records.

Medical text classification focuses on categorizing medical documents or snippets into predefined categories, such as disease types or ICD codes. Pascual et al. [15] utilized BERT for automatic ICD coding, achieving significant improvements over traditional methods. Xu et al. [16] explored multimodal approaches by incorporating both text and image data for medical report classification.

Recent advancements also highlight the integration of domain-specific pre-trained models for these tasks. BioBERT [17] and ClinicalBERT [18] have demonstrated their efficacy in improving the performance of various clinical NLP tasks by incorporating biomedical corpora during pre-training. Additionally, Nerella et al. [19] proposed a transformer-based framework for end-to-end medical entity extraction and classification, showing robust results in clinical datasets.

These studies underscore the importance of domain adaptation and task-specific fine-tuning in achieving state-of-the-art performance in medical information extraction and classification tasks.

In this CHIP evaluation task, we need to extract key information from patient cases first, and then classify cell tumors according to these information.

2.3 Chain-of-Thought

Chain-of-Thought (CoT) prompting, introduced by Wei et al. [20], is a technique that guides Large Language Models (LLMs) to generate intermediate reasoning steps that lead to a final answer. Recent studies have shown that CoT significantly enhances model reasoning capabilities. For instance, Zhou et al. [21] proposed least-to-most prompting, which breaks down complex problems into simpler sub-problems to be solved sequentially. Zhang et al. [22] introduced AutoCoT, an automatic CoT prompting approach that diversifies question samples and generates reasoning chains for demonstrations. In zero-shot contexts,

Kojima et al. [23] used specific phrases (e.g., "let's think in one step") to prompt LLMs to produce effective intermediate steps. Zelikman et al. [24] further refined CoT by generating multiple intermediate steps and selecting those most likely to lead to the correct answer.

These studies underscore the role of CoT in enhancing LLM reasoning, motivating us to integrate CoT-inspired techniques in designing solutions for our evaluation task.

2.4 Parameters-Efficient Optimizations

As Large Language Models (LLMs) grow in parameter size, fully fine-tuning them for downstream tasks becomes increasingly resource-intensive. To address this challenge, several parameter-efficient fine-tuning (PEFT) methods have been developed, allowing pre-trained LLMs to adapt to various tasks efficiently. Three common approaches in PEFT are adapter tuning, prefix tuning, and LoRA.

Adapter methods introduce small task-specific modules within the pretrained model, training only these modules while keeping the rest of the model parameters frozen. Hu et al. [25] proposed LLM-Adapters, a flexible framework for incorporating adapters into LLMs, enabling efficient task-specific adaptation. Prefix Tuning adds task-specific, continuous prefixes to model inputs or hidden layers. Li et al. [26] pioneered this method, optimizing a small, continuous vector to adapt large pre-trained models for new tasks.

LoRA (Low-Rank Adaptation), introduced by Hu et al. [11], approximates the parameter updates of full-rank weight matrices using low-rank matrices, significantly reducing the number of trainable parameters. This method trains only small, learnable matrices while maintaining the model's performance.

In this study, we adopt QLoRA [27], a technique combining low-precision quantization and fine-tuning. QLoRA quantizes pre-trained models to 4-bit precision while introducing learnable low-rank adapter weights. These adapter weights are fine-tuned using backpropagation on the quantized model, achieving efficient and high-fidelity tuning.

3   Methodology

3.1   Model Structure

In this section, we will describe the framework designed for the tasks of lymphoma information extraction and automatic generation of tumor codes. The complete framework, as shown in Fig. 1, is divided into four parts. The first part is about data processing, which includes generating a dictionary of ICD-10 codes and transforming the original data into the input format suitable for large models. The second part is the extraction of text information from patient cases. Mainly based on the text, we extract the lymphoma-related diseases diagnosed in patients and their relevant characteristics (such as types, features, etc.), thus generating <Pathological Diagnosis>. Then, according to <Pathological Diagnosis>, we extract the lymphoma-related diseases diagnosed in patients and their corresponding types to generate the corresponding <Diseases and Their Types>. The third part is to form the data in a fine-tuning input format understandable by large models using <Pathological Diagnosis> and <Diseases and Their Types>generated from the training set. We input these data into ChatGPT for data augmentation and get the data with the same ICD-10 code as the input data. For example, if the ICD-10 code of the input data is C90.1, the ICD-10 code of the data after augmentation is also C90.1. Finally, we use the original data and the data after augmentation to fine-tune the Qwen2.5-14B-Instruct model through LoRA, enabling the model to understand and adapt to our tasks. The fourth part is to first classify the <Pathological Diagnosis> and <Diseases and Their Types> generated from the test set according to ICD-10 codes. We select the top 2 possible major categories according to the list of ICD-10 major categories. Then, we take the list of ICD-10 minor categories composed of all the minor categories in the top 2 major categories as options and input them to the large model to classify the specific ICD-10 minor categories. Then, we generate ICD-O-M codes according to the ICD-10 minor categories. Similarly, we take the list of ICD-O-H codes as options and input them together with <Pathological Diagnosis> and <Diseases and Their Types> to the large model to generate ICD-O-H codes.

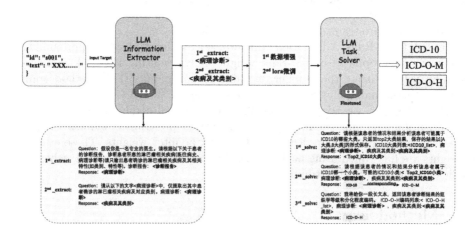

Fig. 1. Overview of our model.

3.2   Task Description

This task is to assign appropriate clinical diagnosis codes for lymphoma cases based on the Tumor Nomenclature and Coding manual compiled by the Shanghai Center for Disease Control and Prevention (1st edition, November 2022). Given a lymphoma case report containing patient details (e.g., demographic information, examination results, diagnoses, and treatments), the task aims to assess the accuracy and efficiency of large models in generating diagnostic codes. By comparing the model's output with human-coded results, this task seeks to evaluate the strengths and limitations of large models and explore their potential for enhancing clinical practice. Output Requirements: The model is expected to extract key information relevant to coding, including: $I = \{Date\ of\ First\ Diagnosis,\ Gender,\ Location\ of\ Tumor,\ Pathological\ Classification,\ etc.\}$ Based on this information, the model should generate the following codes: $O = \{ICD-10,\ ICD-O-M,\ ICD-O-H\}$ This structured output will enable a comprehensive assessment of the model's ability to support tumor registry coding.

3.3   Data Preprocessing

The first stage of the project focuses on data processing, which involves two key tasks: ICD-10 Coding Dictionary Creation, this task requires a thorough understanding of the ICD-10 coding system, including its rules and classification standards. The process involves meticulous organization and validation to ensure the dictionary's accuracy and completeness. A well-constructed ICD-10 dictionary provides essential support for downstream tasks, serving as a reliable reference for disease classification and coding. Raw Data Transformation for Model Input, the second task involves converting raw data into a format compatible with the large model. This process begins with an analysis of key information within the raw data, such as patient details, clinical findings, and diagnostic outcomes. The data is then cleaned and transformed to meet the specific input requirements of the model. By ensuring data consistency and quality, this step establishes a robust foundation for subsequent modeling tasks.

3.4   Textual Information Extraction

The second part of this task primarily focuses on the extraction of text information from patient cases. This process is of great significance as it plays a crucial role in obtaining valuable insights about the patients' conditions. Mainly, we carefully analyze and extract relevant details from the text content of each patient case. Specifically, we zero in on the lymphoma-related diseases that have been diagnosed in the patients. This is not just about identifying the presence of lymphoma but also delving deeper into understanding the specific types of lymphoma involved. For example, it could be Hodgkin's lymphoma or non-Hodgkin's lymphoma, and further differentiating among the various subtypes within these broad categories. In addition to identifying the diseases, we also pay close attention to their relevant characteristics. These characteristics can encompass a wide range of aspects such as the types of lymphoma cells present, the unique features exhibited by the disease, like its growth pattern, how it affects different organs or systems in the body, and any specific symptoms or manifestations that are distinct to that particular type of lymphoma. By comprehensively considering these factors, we are able to generate a more detailed and accurate <Pathological Diagnosis>. Once the <Pathological Diagnosis> has been formulated, our next step is to further extract specific information from it. We extract the lymphoma-related diseases that have been diagnosed in the patients once again, but this time with a particular focus on their corresponding types. This means categorizing the diseases precisely according to the established classification systems for lymphoma. Through this meticulous extraction process, we are then able to generate the corresponding <Diseases and Their Types>, which provides a clear and concise overview of specific lymphoma diseases and their exact types as diagnosed in each patient case. This information will serve as a solid foundation for subsequent analyses and decision-making processes related to the treatment and management of these patients.

3.5 Data Enhancement and Fine-Tuning

The third part of this task is centered around the manipulation and utilization of data to enhance the performance and adaptability of the model for our specific requirements. To begin with, we take the <Pathological Diagnosis> and <Diseases and Their Types> that have been generated from the comprehensive training set. These two elements hold crucial information about the diagnosed conditions and their classifications. Our aim is to transform and organize this data into a fine-tuning input format that can be easily comprehended by large language models. This process involves careful structuring and formatting of the data, ensuring that all the relevant details are presented in a way that aligns with the input expectations of the models. It requires a deep understanding of both the nature of the data we have and the input requirements of the large models to achieve an optimal format. Once we have successfully prepared the data in the appropriate fine-tuning input format, we then proceed to input these data into ChatGPT. The purpose of this step is to carry out data augmentation. ChatGPT, with its powerful language processing capabilities, can analyze the input data and generate additional data that shares similar characteristics. Importantly, we are specifically looking for the data that has the same ICD-10 code as the input data. For instance, if the ICD-10 code of the input data we initially provide is C90.1, then after the data augmentation process within ChatGPT, the ICD-10 code of the newly generated data should also be C90.1. This ensures that the augmented data remains consistent with the original data in terms of the disease classification coding, which is vital for maintaining the accuracy and relevance of our subsequent model fine-tuning. After obtaining the augmented data from ChatGPT, we now have both the original data and the data that has been enhanced through augmentation. The final step in this part of the task is to utilize these two sets of data to fine-tune the Qwen2.5-14B-Instruct model. We employ the LoRA (Low-Rank Adaptation) technique for this fine-tuning process. LoRA allows us to make targeted adjustments to the model's parameters in a more efficient and effective manner. By feeding both the original and augmented data into the model during the fine-tuning process, we are enabling the Qwen2.5-14B-Instruct model to better understand the nuances and patterns within our specific task-related data. This, in turn, helps the model to adapt more effectively to our tasks, ultimately leading to improved performance and more accurate results when dealing with similar types of data in the future (Fig. 2).

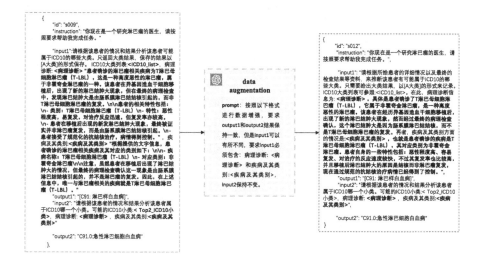

Fig. 2. Examples of our model fine-tuning and prompt.

3.6   Classification and Code Generation

The fourth part of this task entails a series of steps for further classification and code generation based on the data obtained from the test set. Firstly, we focus on the <Pathological Diagnosis> and <Diseases and Their Types> that have been generated from the test set. Our initial action is to classify these according to the ICD-10 codes. The ICD-10 coding system provides a comprehensive framework for categorizing diseases, and by aligning our data with this system, we can better understand and manage the information related to the diagnosed conditions. Once the classification according to ICD-10 codes is underway, we then proceed to select the top 2 possible major categories. This selection is made based on the list of ICD-10 major categories. By identifying these top 2 major categories, we can narrow down our focus and work with a more targeted set of disease classifications that are likely to be relevant to the specific cases we are dealing with. After determining the top 2 major categories, we then take the next step of constructing a list of ICD-10 minor categories. This list is composed of all the minor categories that fall within the top 2 major categories we have just identified. We consider this list of minor categories as options and input them to the large model. The purpose of this input is to enable the large model to classify the specific ICD-10 minor categories accurately. The large model, with its advanced capabilities, can analyze the input data along with the provided options and make more precise classifications within the context of the ICD-10 coding system. Subsequently, once the specific ICD-10 minor categories have been classified by the large model, we then move on to generate ICD-O-M codes according to the identified ICD-10 minor categories. The ICD-O-M codes are crucial for further characterizing the morphological and behavioral aspects of the diseases, and by generating them based on the ICD-10 minor categories, we can provide a more detailed and comprehensive description of the diagnosed conditions. Similarly, we also handle the generation of ICD-O-H codes. We take the list of ICD-O-H codes as options and input them together with the <Pathological Diagnosis> and <Diseases and Their Types> to the large model. The large model then processes this combined input to generate the appropriate ICD-O-H codes. The ICD-O-H codes are significant for indicating the histological grade and degree of differentiation of the diseases, and through this process, we can complete the coding process for a more accurate and detailed representation of the patient's condition.

4   Experiments

4.1   Data Analysis

The dataset consists of 162 lymphoma case reports sourced from published Chinese clinical case studies, divided equally into training (54), test A (54), and test B (54) sets. Test A data is used for model debugging, while Test B is reserved for final evaluation. The data includes detailed patient histories and key attributes such as first diagnosis date, gender, location, pathological classification, and various ICD codes (ICD-10, ICD-O-P, ICD-O-M, ICD-O-H). Patient histories serve as model input, while auxiliary attributes are extracted for coding support without impacting rankings. Model performance is evaluated based on ICD-10, ICD-O-M, and ICD-O-H codes, weighted at 0.3, 0.5, and 0.2, respectively. This structured dataset enables comprehensive assessment of the model's capability in lymphoma diagnostic coding (Table 1).

Table 1. The dataset contains a total of 162 case reports related to lymphoma. The specific categorization is shown in the table.

Type	Number
Train	54
test A	54
test B	54

4.2   Parameter Settings

During the training process, we used the LoRA framework to partially tune the parameters of the Qwen2.5-14B-Instruct model for a total of 5 epochs of training. The learning rate was set to 2×10^{-4} and the batch_size was 2. In addition, the parameters used by LoRA in the fine-tuning included the LoRA_rank Of 64, the LoRA_alpha of 16, and the LoRA_dropout of 0.05. The parameters of the specific model are shown in Table 2.

Table 2. Experimental parameter settings.

Qwen2.5-14B-Instruct+ LoRA	learning rate	2×10^{-4}
	epoch	5
	batch_size	2
	LoRA_rank	64
	LoRA_alpha	16
	LoRA_dropout	0.05

4.3   Explanation of Scoring Rules

In this task, the final ranking scores were calculated based on the accuracy of the model in the automatic code generation section. Each tumor code contains ICD-10 coding, ICD-O-M morphology coding and behavioral coding, and ICD-O-H histological grade and differentiation coding, and different weights are given to different parts in the final calculation, including 0.3 for ICD-10 coding, 0.5 for ICD-O-M morphology coding and behavioral coding, and 0.2 for ICD-O-H histological grade and differentiation coding. The final ranking score is the sum of the weighted accuracy of all parts, and the average of the weighted scores of the model in all samples is its final ranking score, which is calculated by the following formula:

$$\text{Accuracy-icd-10} = \frac{\text{Number of samples with correct ICD-10 codes}}{\text{Total sample size}} \quad (1)$$

$$\text{Accuracy-icd-o-m} = \frac{\text{Number of samples with correct ICD-O-M codes}}{\text{Total sample size}} \quad (2)$$

$$\text{Accuracy-icd-o-h} = \frac{\text{Number of samples with correct ICD-O-H codes}}{\text{Total sample size}} \quad (3)$$

$$\text{Accuracy} = 0.3 \times \text{Accuracy-icd-10} + 0.5 \times \text{Accuracy-icd-o-m} + 0.2 \times \text{Accuracy-icd-o-h} \quad (4)$$

4.4   Results Analysis and Case Study

Table 3. Results of different methods and different base models

Model	Method	Accuracy
Qwen2.5-0.5B-Instruct	direct extraction and direct classification	10.91
LLama-7B	direct extraction and direct classification	25.53
Qwen2.5-7B-Instruct	direct extraction and direct classification	27.53
Qwen2.5-14B-Instruct	direct extraction and direct classification	32.04
Qwen2.5-14B-Instruct	hierarchical extraction and direct classification	51.30
Qwen2.5-14B-Instruct	hierarchical extraction, hierarchical classification	69.76
Fine-tuning Qwen2.5-14B-Instruct	hierarchical extraction, hierarchical classification	85.00

Table 3 presents the results of our method on the test B, illustrating how various model improvements impact performance.

We observe that the classification accuracy increases in tandem with the growth of the model's parameter count, which aligns with an established objective principle. However, our servers have limitations in supporting the fine - tuning of larger models. As a result, our experiments have only managed to yield results with a 14 - billion - parameter model. We also experimented with the Llama - 7B model. When the model setups had the same number of parameters, Llama - 7B did not perform as effectively as Qwen - 7B. We hypothesize that this disparity may be attributed to Qwen's superior adaptability to Chinese - language application scenarios.

1. Direct Extraction and Classification: Using Qwen2.5-14B-Instruct to directly extract information from patient cases and classify yields a score of 32.04%. This lower score is attributed to significant noise introduced during the direct extraction of disease information, which negatively affects lymphoma coding accuracy, resulting in confusing outputs.
2. Hierarchical Extraction: By first extracting <Pathological Diagnosis> followed by <Disease and its Category>, and then using this refined information for classification, the score improves to 51.30%. This method reduces noise from the case data, and the <Disease and its Category> derived from

<Pathological Diagnosis> provides a more precise description of the patient's disease.

3. Hierarchical Extraction and Classification: This method involves generating <Pathological Diagnosis> and <Diseases and their Types> from the test set, followed by a two-step classification process, the score improves to 69.76%. First, ICD-10 broad categories are predicted, selecting the top two candidates. Then, subcategories within these top two are classified to produce specific ICD-10 codes.

4. Fine-Tuning with Enhanced Training Data: Fine-tuning the model using augmented training data significantly improves task-specific adaptation, the score improves to 85.00%. For instance,3 the original model often misclassified T-lymphoblastic leukemia/lymphoma as C85.9, C91.9, or C84.4, when the correct code is C91.0. After fine-tuning, the model correctly identifies this subtype, having learned the proper categorization from the training set. Similarly, Mucosa-Associated Lymphoid Tissue Extranodal Marginal Zone Lymphoma (MALT Lymphoma), initially misclassified as C85.1, is accurately categorized as C88.4 post fine-tuning. This occurs because the model lacks precise knowledge regarding the categories to which the two diseases belong. Consequently, it classifies them in the most similar manner based on the information available in its internal database, yet this results in misclassification. In fact, these two examples are quite similar within the training set. The model, through fine - tuning, learns that, for instance, the CID - 10 code for a particular disease should be assigned to a specific category. It retains this information, and the next time it encounters a similar instance, it is able to classify it accurately.

```
{
    "id": "s120",
    "response": "根据提供的病理诊断信息，可以提取出
以下患者确诊的淋巴瘤相关疾病及其类别：\n\n- 疾病名称:
T-淋巴母细胞白血病/淋巴瘤 (T-LBL/T-ALL) \n- 类别: 淋巴
母细胞型\n\n这是一种高度恶性的淋巴瘤，主要涉及T细胞
的异常增生。"
},
```

```
{
    "id": "s128",
    "response": "根据提供的病理诊断信息，患者确诊的淋巴瘤相关疾
病及其类别如下：\n\n- **疾病名称**：胃黏膜相关淋巴组织 (MALT) 淋
巴瘤\n- **类别**：小B细胞性淋巴瘤，属于结外边缘区淋巴瘤的一种\n\n
这表明该患者的具体淋巴瘤类型是胃MALT淋巴瘤，它是一种低度恶性的
B细胞淋巴瘤，且属于结外边缘区淋巴瘤范畴。"
},
```

```
微调前:
C85.9非霍奇金淋巴瘤NOS、C91.9淋
巴样白血病NOS
C84.4粘膜相关淋巴结结外边缘区
[MALT] (B细胞) ,
微调后:
C91.0急性淋巴细胞白血病[ALL]
```

```
微调前:
C85.1细胞淋巴瘤NOS,
微调后:
C88.4粘膜相关淋巴结结外边缘区[MALT] (B细胞) 淋巴瘤
```

Fig. 3. Case study for fine-tuning.

5   Conclusion

This section details a framework for lymphoma information extraction and automatic tumor code generation. Comprising four parts: (1) Data processing involves creating an ICD-10 code dictionary and formatting original data for large models. (2) Text information extraction from patient cases to obtain lymphoma-related diseases and characteristics, generating <Pathological Diagnosis> and then <Disease and its Category>. (3) Using <Pathological Diagnosis> and <Diseases and Their Types> from the training set to form fine-tuning input data, augmenting it via ChatGPT with the same ICD-10 code, and fine-tuning the Qwen2.5-14B-Instruct model with original and augmented data. (4) Classifying <Pathological Diagnosis> and <Diseases and Their Types> from the test set by ICD-10 codes, selecting top 2 major categories, using their minor categories for further classification, and generating ICD-O-M and ICD-O-H codes. Experimental results show that the framework performs well in the domain of medical information extraction and medical disease classification with high accuracy. Finally, our model is ranked fifth in the test set evaluation in the task of lymphoma information extraction and automatic tumor coding generation for CHIP 2024.

References

1. Zong, H., et al.: Advancing chinese biomedical text mining with community challenges. J. Biomed. Inform. 104716 (2024)
2. Yang, A., et al.: Qwen2 technical report. arXiv preprint arXiv:2407.10671 (2024)
3. Liu, J., Shen, D., Zhang, Y., Dolan, B., Carin, L., Chen, W.: What makes good in-context examples for GPT-3? arXiv preprint arXiv:2101.06804 (2021)
4. Touvron, H., et al. LLaMA: open and efficient foundation language models. arXiv preprint arXiv:2302.13971 (2023)
5. Chowdhery, A., et al.: PaLM: scaling language modeling with pathways. arXiv preprint arXiv:2204.02311 (2022)
6. Du, Z., et al.: GLM: general language model pretraining with autoregressive blank infilling. arXiv preprint arXiv:2103.10360 (2021)
7. Zeng, A., et al. GLM-130B: an open bilingual pre-trained model. arXiv preprint arXiv:2210.02414, 2022
8. Singhal, K., et al.: Towards expert-level medical question answering with large language models. arXiv preprint arXiv:2305.09617 (2023)
9. Li, Y., Li, Z., Zhang, K., Dan, R., Zhang, Y.: ChatDoctor: a medical chat model fine-tuned on llama model using medical domain knowledge. arXiv preprint arXiv:2303.14070 (2023)
10. Xiong, H., et al.: DoctorGLM: fine-tuning your Chinese doctor is not a herculean task. arXiv preprint arXiv:2304.01097 (2023)
11. Hu, E.J., et al.: LoRA: low-rank adaptation of large language models. arXiv preprint arXiv:2106.09685 (2021)
12. Wang, H., et al.: Huatuo: tuning llama model with Chinese medical knowledge. arXiv preprint arXiv:2304.06975 (2023)
13. An, Y., Xia, X., Chen, X., Fang-Xiang, W., Wang, J.: Chinese clinical named entity recognition via multi-head self-attention based biLSTM-CRF. Artif. Intell. Med. **127**, 102282 (2022)
14. Singhal, A., Simmons, M., Zhiyong, L.: Text mining for precision medicine: automating disease-mutation relationship extraction from biomedical literature. J. Am. Med. Inform. Assoc. **23**(4), 766–772 (2016)

15. Pascual, D., Luck, S., Wattenhofer, R.: Towards BERT-based automatic ICD coding: Limitations and opportunities. arXiv preprint arXiv:2104.06709 (2021)
16. Xu, K., et al. Multimodal machine learning for automated ICD coding. In: Machine Learning for Healthcare Conference, pp. 197–215. PMLR (2019)
17. Lee, J., et al.: BioBERT: a pre-trained biomedical language representation model for biomedical text mining. Bioinformatics **36**(4), 1234–1240 (2020)
18. Huang, K., Altosaar, J., Ranganath, R.: ClinicalBERT: modeling clinical notes and predicting hospital readmission. arXiv preprint arXiv:1904.05342 (2019)
19. Nerella, S., et al. Transformers in healthcare: a survey. arXiv preprint arXiv:2307.00067 (2023)
20. Wei, J., et al.: Chain-of-thought prompting elicits reasoning in large language models. Adv. Neural. Inf. Process. Syst. **35**, 24824–24837 (2022)
21. Zhou, D., et al. Least-to-most prompting enables complex reasoning in large language models. arXiv preprint arXiv:2205.10625 (2022)
22. Zhang, Z., Zhang, A., Li, M., Smola, A.: Automatic chain of thought prompting in large language models. arXiv preprint arXiv:2210.03493 (2022)
23. Kojima, T., Gu, S.S., Reid, M., Matsuo, Y., Iwasawa, Y.: Large language models are zero-shot reasoners. Adv. Neural. Inf. Process. Syst. **35**, 22199–22213 (2022)
24. Zelikman, E., Yuhuai, W., Jesse, M., Goodman, N.: STAR: bootstrapping reasoning with reasoning. Adv. Neural. Inf. Process. Syst. **35**, 15476–15488 (2022)
25. Hu, Z., et al.: LLM-adapters: an adapter family for parameter-efficient fine-tuning of large language models. arXiv preprint arXiv:2304.01933 (2023)
26. Li, X.L., Liang, P.: Prefix-tuning: optimizing continuous prompts for generation. arXiv preprint arXiv:2101.00190 (2021)
27. Dettmers, T., Pagnoni, A., Holtzman, A., Zettlemoyer, L.: QLoRA: efficient fine-tuning of quantized LLMs. arXiv preprint arXiv:2305.14314 (2023)

Typical Case Diagnosis Consistency

Benchmark of the Typical Case Diagnosis Consistency Evaluation Task in CHIP 2024

Zehua Wang[1], Hui Zong[2], Yang Feng[3], ZhaoRong Teng[3], Jun Yan[3], Shujia Jiang[3], and Buzhou Tang[1,4(✉)]

[1] Harbin Institute of Technology (Shenzhen), Shenzhen 518055, Guangdong, China
tangbuzhou@hit.edu.cn
[2] West China Hospital, Sichuan University, Chengdu 610041, Sichuan, China
[3] Yidu Cloud, Beijing 100000, China
[4] Pengcheng Laboratory, Shenzhen 518055, Guangdong, China

Abstract. This article mainly introduces the medical benchmark in the Typical Case Diagnosis Consistency Evaluation Task released at the CHIP 2024 conference (see http://www.cips-chip.org.cn/2024/eval3 for details). Unlike other existing benchmarks, this benchmark is built on the basis of real medical record information screened manually and has been strictly reviewed by medical experts to maximize the diagnostic ability of large models in real clinical environments. In addition, this benchmark not only covers a variety of complex cases, but also fully considers the diversity of cases and the authenticity of diagnostic scenarios, providing an important reference for evaluating the generalization ability and practical application potential of medical large models.

Keywords: Typical Case Diagnosis Consistency · Large language models · Benchmark for medicine

1 Introduction

In recent years, with the rapid development of general big models, medical large models have also achieved remarkable results in various tasks. It can be seen that medical large models not only have rich expert knowledge, but also perform well in many evaluation tasks such as medical text generation, medical information extraction, and question-answering systems, and their development trend is thriving. Many evaluation benchmarks have been established for the medical field, such as medical named entity recognition [10], relationship extraction [6], and medical literature PICOS identificationn [12], but there are relatively few diagnostic evaluations based on real data, especially high-quality evaluation data for evaluating the diagnostic ability of diagnostic large models is even more scarce.

To fill this gap and accelerate the practical application of medical large models, we have built a new evaluation benchmark based on real data. This benchmark integrates the diagnostic information of many common diseases, covering a

© The Author(s), under exclusive license to Springer Nature Singapore Pte Ltd. 2025
Y. Zhang et al. (Eds.): CHIP 2024, CCIS 2458, pp. 149–157, 2025.
https://doi.org/10.1007/978-981-96-4298-4_13

wide range of categories such as common diseases, chronic diseases, and rare diseases, while retaining key content in real clinical scenarios, including chief complaints, current medical history, past history, family history, personal history, marital history, auxiliary examinations, specialist examinations, physical examinations, laboratory examinations, and disease diagnosis. By accurately restoring the decision-making process of doctors diagnosing diseases, the benchmark fully simulates the complex and changeable diagnostic conditions and constraints in real medical scenarios.

In addition, in order to improve the authority and medical adaptability of the benchmark, we introduced a team of medical experts in the benchmark construction process to strictly review and calibrate each medical record data to ensure its clinical authenticity and diagnostic accuracy. At the same time, the benchmark also designed a set of multi-dimensional evaluation indicators, including accuracy, recall rate, F1 score, and multi-disease coverage, to comprehensively evaluate the diagnostic capabilities ofmedical large models from multiple angles.

The launch of this benchmark not only fills the gap in real medical record diagnosis evaluation, but also provides a reliable basis for the performance verification of medical large models in practical applications, and helps the further development and promotion of medical artificial intelligence technology. In the future, we plan to expand the benchmark to more disease types and more complex clinical scenarios to continuously promote the technical innovation and application of medical large models.

2   Benchmark for Medical Large Model

These benchmarks simulate real-world clinical scenarios to measure the model's ability to understand medical knowledge, perform clinical reasoning, and provide accurate medical advice. There are already many benchmarks that measure the different capabilities of the model: MIMIC-III and MIMIC-IV datasets [1] evaluate the model's abilities in clinical data processing, report generation, clinical summarization, and patient outcome prediction through extensive electronic health records (EHRs); BioASQ [9] and PubMedQA [4] datasets focus on the model's understanding and question-answering capabilities in biomedical literature. MedQA [3] and MedMCQA [7] datasets evaluate the model's medical knowledge and reasoning skills through multiple-choice question formats. MMLU-Med [8] which is the medical and biological subset of MMLU measures the model's language understanding capabilities in specific domains. In addition, many multimodal benchmarks further examine the ability of large medical models to handle tasks in different modalities: VQA-RAD [5], the first manually constructed dataset where clinicians asked naturally occurring questions about radiology images and provided reference answers. PATH-VQA [2] which contains 32,799 question-answer pairs of 7 categories, is generated from 4,998 images. PMC-VQA [11], which contains 227k VQA pairs of 149k images that cover various modalities or diseases. Majority of questions in this dataset are open-ended, posing great challenges for the medical VQA research. Together, these datasets form a multidimensional assessment framework, helping researchers to comprehensively understand and enhance the performance of medical large models in a variety of medical tasks.

Further research is needed to establish more standardized, universal benchmarks for medical large models, as this will facilitate the comparison of different models and accelerate the adoption of AI technologies in healthcare. Benchmarking also includes external validation, where models are tested on real-world clinical data or data from different institutions to assess their generalization ability. This helps ensure that models perform reliably across diverse clinical environments.

3   Diagnostic Consistency Benchmark

The Diagnostic Consistency Benchmark is designed to rigorously evaluate the diagnostic reasoning and decision-making capabilities of large-scale medical models. By leveraging real-world clinical data and ensuring a high level of data quality through expert review, this benchmark provides a comprehensive framework for assessing model performance in realistic clinical scenarios. It aims to bridge the gap between academic research and practical medical applications, offering valuable insights into the strengths and limitations of current diagnostic models. This benchmark not only highlights the importance of accurate and consistent diagnostic predictions but also sets a standard for future advancements in medical AI evaluation.

This benchmark evaluates the model through an indefinite multiple-choice QA. Specifically, the patient information is set as the question and the diagnosis result is the answer. Examples of single-choice and multiple-choice questions are shown in Fig. 1 and Fig. 2. Each instance consists of the following fields: **id** is the unique identifier of the data, which is used to ensure the uniqueness of the data; **text** contains detailed information of the medical record, including basic information of the patient, chief complaint, current medical history, personal history, family history, past history, physical examination and laboratory tests, etc.; **question_type** refers to the type of question, which can be single-choice or multiple-choice; **options** provides disease options, expressed in key-value pair format; **answer_idx** is the index of the correct answer, in list format, which can contain one or more correct options. These fields together describe a case and its corresponding diagnostic multiple-choice question, providing complete case information and assessment objectives.

The benchmark contains 4239 cases in total and two rounds of data splitting are performed for this task. The division of each data format and its distribution in the two rounds of tasks are shown in Table 1. Next we describe the process of building this benchmark and analyzing it.

{
"text": "个人信息: 男性, 14 岁。\n主诉: 反复自杀 2 年, 沉迷手机, 情绪不稳 1 年余。\n现病史: 患儿近 2 年有多次自伤自杀史, 如跳楼、跳水、吞服蟑螂丸等。2020 年 2 月疫情期间, 患儿不愿上网课, 沉迷手机, 睡眠差, 脾气暴躁, 砸家里门窗、电器, 与父亲对打, 生活懒散, 间断上学。曾在外院就诊, 诊断不详, 拒绝服药。近 1 年来间断上学, 每次上学只能坚持几天, 2021 年 9 月 19 日患儿喝农药后被送至医院抢救, 9 月 25 日出院, 建议至本院就诊。9 月 26 日患儿住院治疗, 诊断为 "通常在童年和青少年期发病的行为和情绪障碍", 给予丙戊酸镁和喹硫平口服治疗, 11 天后患儿表示愿意回家上学, 家属办理自动出院。出院后患儿仍脾气大, 在家打父亲, 砸门, 玩游戏, 不愿上学, 较任性, 家属难以管理。\n既往史: 3 岁时因吐词不清行舌部手术, 6 岁时因车祸左大腿骨折手术治疗。否认药物过敏史, 否认炎、结核等传染病病史。\n个人史: 自小生长发育正常, 第一胎, 足月剖腹产; 6 岁时父母离异, 随父亲生活, 母亲每年探视一两次, 父亲未再婚, 母亲已再婚, 初中文化, 病前性格外向, 无烟酒等嗜好。\n家族史: 阳性, 患儿大姑有精神异常史, 服农药死亡, 具体不详。\n体格检查: 全身散发皮疹, 无破溃, 左腿可见一长约 15cm 手术瘢痕, 双侧瞳孔等大等圆, 直径 3mm, 心肺听诊无异常, 神经系统检查未见阳性病理征。\n检查检验: 颅脑 CT 平扫未见明显异常。胸部正位片示两肺、心膈未见明显异常, 血常规, 肝功能、电解质、血糖、血脂、甲状腺功能未见明显异常。甲肝抗体、乙肝抗体、丙肝抗体、梅毒抗体、HIV 抗体、尿毒品均为阴性。精神状况检查: 意识清楚, 定向力完整, 接触交谈被动, 问话能答, 对答切题, 否认幻觉、错觉及综合障碍, 思维联想速度可, 存在牵连观念, 情绪不稳, 自诉烦躁, 在家跟奶奶及父亲难以沟通, 看不起奶奶及父亲, 自我评价低, 觉得不如其他人, 因为心情不好, 自卑所以沉迷网络, 觉得自己拖了班级后腿, 所以不想去上学, 情感反应尚协调, 生活懒散, 智力、记忆力可, 自知力不全。",
"diagnosis": "通常在童年和青少年期发病的行为和情绪障碍",
"id": "1499668",
"question_type": "单选题",
"answer": ["通常在童年和青少年期发病的行为和情绪障碍"],
"options": {"A": "通常在童年和青少年期发病的行为和情绪障碍", "B": "精神分裂症", "C": "抑郁症", "D": "双相情感障碍" },
"answer_idx": ["A"]
}

Fig. 1. Single choice case example.

{
"text": "个人信息\n\n- 年龄: 48 岁\n- 性别: 女\n\n主诉\n\n\n发现直肠癌及肝转移癌 6 个月。\n\n现病史\n\n患者于 2022 年 10 月体检行腹部 B 超发现肝占位, 完善腹部 CT 后考虑直肠占位、肝占位, 行后电子肠镜及病理检查提示腺癌, 部分为黏液腺癌。就诊于外院, 行 COIBx 方案化疗 10 个周期, 期间无明显不适。2023 年 4 月 10 日入院后复查腹部 CT 示直肠上段肠壁增厚, 符合直肠癌; 肝内多发转移瘤, 同时肿瘤标志物升高。2023 年 6 月 12 日上腹部 MRI 示肝内多发占位, 考虑转移瘤, 胆囊结石。2023 年 6 月 19 日全腹部血管增强 CT 示肝介入治疗术后改变, 肝多发病灶较前变化不著, 直肠上段肠壁增厚, 符合直肠癌; 肝钙化灶; 胆囊结石; 肝右动脉起源异位。\n\n既往史\n\n\n无肿瘤相关病史家族史及传染病史。\n\n个人史\n\n\n无特殊。\n\n六. 家族史**\n\n无肿瘤家族史。\n\n体格检查\n\n\n无。\n\n检查检验\n\n- 2022 年 10 月 9 日化疗前上腹部 MRI: 肝脏多发大小不等结节及肿块影, 双叶多段分布, 大者约 8.4 cm×8.1 cm, 考虑肝转移瘤。- 2022 年 10 月 10 日直肠 MRI: 直肠上段肠壁不均匀增厚形成肿物, 考虑恶性, 侵及肠壁全层, 建议结合临床及镜检, 病变周围, 骶前, 直肠系膜筋膜内多发肿大淋巴结, 警惕转移, 建议追随。- 2022 年 10 月 11 日病理检查: 直肠活检腺癌, 中分化。\n- 2023 年 4 月 10 日入院后腹部 CT: 直肠上段肠壁增厚, 符合直肠癌, 肝内多发转移瘤, 脾大约 58 mm×47 mm。\n- 2023 年 6 月 12 日上腹部 MRI: 肝内多发占位, 结合病史, 考虑转移瘤、胆囊结石。\n- 2023 年 6 月 19 日全腹部血管增强 CT: 肝介入治疗术后改变, 肝多发病灶较前变化不著, 直肠上段肠壁增厚, 符合直肠癌; 肝钙化灶; 胆囊结石; 肝右动脉起源异位。\n- 肿瘤标志物: TPS 487.219 U/L, CEA 215.00 ng/ml, CA72-4 154.00 U/ml; CA-199 为 2.06 U/ml, CEA 为 35.09 ng/ml。",
"diagnosis": "肝继发恶性肿瘤; 直肠恶性肿瘤; 胆囊结石",
"id": "1496982", "question_type": "多选题",
"answer": ["肝继发恶性肿瘤", "直肠恶性肿瘤", "胆囊结石"],
"options": {"A": "肝继发恶性肿瘤", "B": "直肠恶性肿瘤", "C": "胆囊结石", "D": "肝血管瘤", "E": "肝囊肿", "F": "结肠癌", "G": "胰腺" },
"answer_idx": ["A", "B", "C"]
}

Fig. 2. Multiple choice case example.

Table 1. The overview of the benchmark.

Form	Round 1	Round 2	All
Single	2365	179	2544
Multiple	874	821	1695

3.1 Data Source

The data for the diagnostic consistency benchmark is primarily sourced from the Chinese Medical Care Repository[1]. This repository provides a diverse collection of real-world medical cases, reflecting typical scenarios encountered in clinical practice. It includes cases covering a variety of diseases, patient demographics, and clinical complexities, making it a reliable foundation for evaluating the diagnostic capabilities of large medical models.

3.2 Data Processing Process

To ensure the quality and clinical relevance of the benchmark, the data underwent a rigorous multi-step processing procedure:

1. **Data Collection:** Medical cases were systematically selected from the Chinese Medical Care Repository.
2. **Feature Extraction:** Essential information was extracted from each case using the Yidu AI medical model. This process focused on key components such as:Chief complaints,Present illness history, Past medical history, Family history, Personal history, Marital and reproductive history, Auxiliary examinations, Specialized physical examinations, General physical examinations, Laboratory tests and Disease diagnoses.
3. **Quality Review:** We introduced medical experts to conduct this re-review of the medical records in the previous step. Specifically, Anomalous cases, including those with incomplete or inconsistent information, were carefully reviewed and excluded. Additionally, cases where the model-extracted features did not align with the original records were filtered out. Furthermore, cases relying on imaging data, such as X-rays or CT scans, were removed to maintain the focus on text-based diagnostic scenarios.
4. **Question Generation:** The process involved constructing questions designed to test diagnostic reasoning and categorizing responses using GPT-based models into three groups: fully correct answers, partially correct answers (e.g., for multiple-choice questions where only some correct options were selected), and incorrect answers (where any wrong selection was made).
5. **Final Selection:** The cases that met the criteria for diagnostic consistency and completeness were included in the benchmark dataset. By the way, We will mix in 10% incorrect and partially correct questions to avoid objectivity issues.

3.3 Data Distribution

The benchmark dataset is structured to provide a balanced and comprehensive evaluation environment. It includes a wide range of diseases and an even distribution of diagnostic complexity and its distribution is shown in Figs. 3, 4 and 5.

---

[1] https://www.yiigle.com/Journal/Detail/185.

The dataset is designed to capture the diversity of real-world clinical scenarios and it involves 6458 types of diseases. The disease distribution highlights the prevalence of both chronic conditions, such as Type 2 diabetes and hypertension, and acute illnesses, such as lung infections, providing a realistic spectrum of diagnostic challenges. As shown in Fig. 3, the top five most common diseases in the dataset are Type 2 diabetes, lung infections, coronary artery disease, hypoproteinemia, and hypertension, with Type 2 diabetes being the most frequently represented condition.

In terms of patient demographics, the dataset includes cases spanning multiple age groups. As shown in Fig. 4, the majority of the cases are concentrated in the 19–65 age range, with age groups 19–35, 36–50, and 51–65 collectively accounting for a significant portion of the data. Pediatric cases (0–18 years) and geriatric cases (66 years and older) are also represented, though their proportions are relatively smaller, ensuring a balanced but diverse age distribution.

Regarding gender representation, the dataset achieves a near-equal balance between male and female patients. Shown in Fig. 5, Male cases slightly outnumber female cases, with males constituting approximately 53.1% of the dataset and females accounting for 46.9%. This balanced gender distribution ensures that diagnostic models are evaluated equitably across both genders.

The dataset also provides varied text lengths for clinical records, reflecting the differences in complexity and detail among cases. See Fig. 6, the text length distribution shows that most records fall within the range of 500 to 1500 characters, with a minority of cases being either significantly shorter or longer. This variability ensures that models are tested on both concise and detailed medical histories.

Overall, the dataset's balanced representation of diseases, patient demographics, and record complexity makes it a robust benchmark for evaluating the diagnostic capabilities of medical AI models.

3.4   Limitations

While the diagnostic consistency benchmark represents a significant step forward in evaluating medical AI models, it has certain limitations:

- **Dependency on Textual Data:** The benchmark exclusively relies on textual data, which may not capture the full scope of clinical diagnostics that often depend on imaging data, such as radiology or pathology images.
- **Generalization Challenges:** The dataset's focus on text-based information might limit its applicability to multimodal diagnostic systems that integrate text and visual inputs.
- **Data Coverage:** Despite its diversity, the dataset may not fully represent all rare diseases or atypical clinical cases encountered in real-world settings.
- **Simplified Scenarios:** The use of multiple-choice and single-choice questions may oversimplify some aspects of clinical decision-making, which often involves nuanced reasoning and contextual judgment.

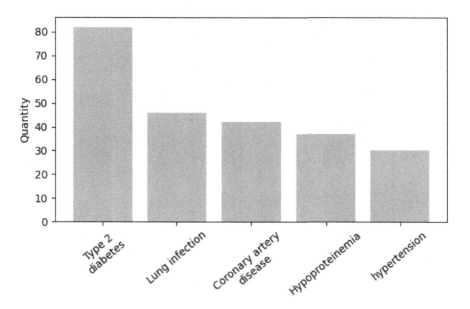

Fig. 3. Distribution of the top 5 disease types.

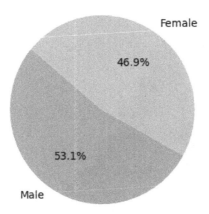

Fig. 4. Gender Ratio.

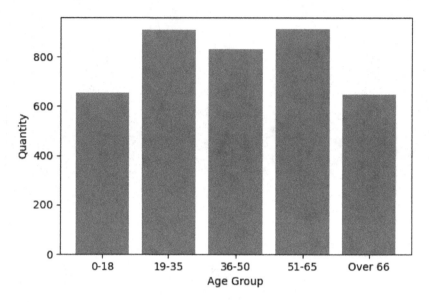

Fig. 5. Age Distribution.

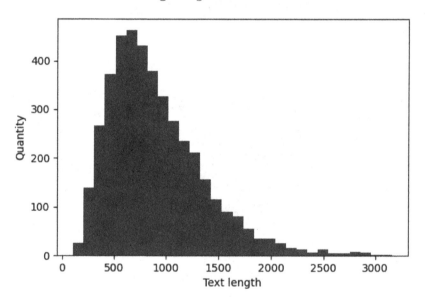

Fig. 6. Distribution of medical record text length.

Despite these limitations, the benchmark provides a robust platform for evaluating diagnostic capabilities and sets the stage for future improvements in medical AI evaluation methodologies.

4   Conclusion

This article introduces in detail the evaluation benchmark used in the CHIP 2024 Typical Case Diagnosis Consistency Evaluation Task. The benchmark is constructed with real case data and has undergone multiple rounds of processing and review by medical experts. Although it still has limitations such as single and data coverage, the benchmark integrates the diagnosis and medical records of many common diseases, and provides a reliable basis for comprehensively and objectively evaluating the diagnostic capabilities of medical large models by accurately restoring the decision-making process of doctors in diagnosing diseases.

References

1. Harutyunyan, H., Khachatrian, H., Kale, D.C., Ver Steeg, G., Galstyan, A.: Multitask learning and benchmarking with clinical time series data. Sci. Data **6**(1), 96 (2019)
2. He, X., Zhang, Y., Mou, L., Xing, E., Xie, P.: PathVQA: 30000+ questions for medical visual question answering. arXiv preprint arXiv:2003.10286 (2020)
3. Jin, D., Pan, E., Oufattole, N., Weng, W.H., Fang, H., Szolovits, P.: What disease does this patient have? A large-scale open domain question answering dataset from medical exams. Appl. Sci. **11**(14), 6421 (2021)
4. Jin, Q., Dhingra, B., Liu, Z., Cohen, W.W., Lu, X.: PubMedQA: a dataset for biomedical research question answering. arXiv preprint arXiv:1909.06146 (2019)
5. Lau, J.J., Gayen, S., Ben Abacha, A., Demner-Fushman, D.: A dataset of clinically generated visual questions and answers about radiology images. Sci. Data (2018). https://doi.org/10.1038/sdata.2018.251
6. Li, Z., et al.: CHIP2022 shared task overview: medical causal entity relationship extraction. In: China Health Information Processing Conference, pp. 51–56. Springer (2022)
7. Pal, A., Umapathi, L.K., Sankarasubbu, M.: MedMCQA: a large-scale multi-subject multi-choice dataset for medical domain question answering. In: Conference on Health, Inference, and Learning, pp. 248–260. PMLR (2022)
8. Singhal, K., et al.: Large language models encode clinical knowledge. arXiv preprint arXiv:2212.13138 (2022)
9. Tsatsaronis, G., et al.: An overview of the BIOASQ large-scale biomedical semantic indexing and question answering competition. BMC Bioinform. **16**, 1–28 (2015)
10. Zhang, C., Li, Y., Zhang, K., Zan, H.: CMF-NERD: Chinese medical few-shot named entity recognition dataset with state-of-the-art evaluation. In: China Health Information Processing Conference, pp. 87–97. Springer (2023)
11. Zhang, X., Wu, C., Zhao, Z., Lin, W., Zhang, Y., Wang, Y., Xie, W.: PMC-VQA: visual instruction tuning for medical visual question answering (2023)
12. Zong, H., Yin, K., Tong, Y., Ma, Z., Xu, J., Tang, B.: Overview of CHIP 2023 shared task 5: medical literature PICOS identification. In: China Health Information Processing Conference, pp. 159–165. Springer (2023)

Overview of the Typical Case Diagnosis Consistency Evaluation Task in CHIP 2024

Zehua Wang[1], Hui Zong[2], Yang Feng[3], ZhaoRong Teng[3], Jun Yan[3], Shujia Jiang[3], and Buzhou Tang[1,4(✉)]

[1] Harbin Institute of Technology (Shenzhen), Shenzhen 518055, Guangdong, China
tangbuzhou@hit.edu.cn
[2] West China Hospital, Sichuan University, Chengdu 610041, Sichuan, China
[3] Yidu Cloud, Beijing 100000, China
[4] Pengcheng Laboratory, Shenzhen 518055, Guangdong, China

Abstract. This paper presents an overview of Typical Case Diagnosis Consistency Evaluation Task in CHIP 2024 Conference. (http://www.cips-chip.org.cn/2024/eval3) This shared task integrates diagnostic medical record information for a variety of common diseases and aims to conduct a comprehensive and monitored evaluation of the diagnostic capabilities of large medical models by simulating the decision-making process of doctors in diagnosing diseases. Numerous teams from both industry and academia actively participated in the shared tasks, with the leading teams achieving remarkable test results. This paper provides a detailed overview of the tasks, datasets, evaluation metrics, and the top-performing solution. Finally, it summarizes the techniques employed and the evaluation results of the diverse approaches explored by the participating teams.

Keywords: Typical Case Diagnosis Consistency · Large language models · Medical natural language processing

1 Introduction

In recent years, alongside the rapid development of general large models, medical large models have also achieved excellent results across various tasks. It is evident that medical large models possess sufficient expert knowledge and have performed very well in many evaluation tasks, indicating the thriving progress of medical large models. Currently, many medical-related NLP tasks have established evaluation tasks, but medical diagnosis tasks based on typical medical records still lack a complete evaluation task and set of indicators.

To continuously improve the application of medical large models in real clinical scenarios and accelerate the implementation of artificial intelligence technology (especially medical large models), we have launched a diagnostic consistency evaluation task based on real medical records. This task integrates diagnostic

© The Author(s), under exclusive license to Springer Nature Singapore Pte Ltd. 2025
Y. Zhang et al. (Eds.): CHIP 2024, CCIS 2458, pp. 158–165, 2025.
https://doi.org/10.1007/978-981-96-4298-4_14

information for a variety of common diseases and aims to comprehensively and objectively evaluate the diagnostic capabilities of medical large models by accurately restoring the decision-making process of doctors in diagnosing diseases. This task has the following characteristics:

- **Authenticity:** The medical record-related information includes routine basic details, chief complaints, medical history, past history, as well as laboratory tests and examinations, reflecting real clinical medical diagnoses.
- **Wide Disease Coverage:** The medical records encompass a range of common diseases across various medical specialties, providing a better assessment of the model's ability to handle the comprehensive nature of medical practice across multiple fields.
- **Comprehensive Evaluation:** The task includes both single-choice and multiple-choice questions. The multiple-choice questions cover primary diagnoses, related past diseases, and complications, offering a deep and comprehensive evaluation with a certain level of challenge.

The Typical Case Diagnosis Consistency Evaluation Task has garnered significant attention from both industry and academia. A lot of teams have participated in various tracks of the shared task. In this paper, we provide an overview of the shared task, highlight the winning teams and their methodologies, and discuss potential directions for future research.

2   Related Work

2.1   Medical Large Model

Medical large models are trained or fine-turned at general large models on amounts of complex medical data, including but not limited to medical images, patient health records, genomic sequences, and more. These models leverage the power of large-scale datasets and cutting-edge machine learning techniques to enhance the efficiency and accuracy of medical diagnoses, treatment planning, and personalized medicine. There are many medical large models trained on different the training corpus sources. One well-known model is **Med-PaLM** [15], a large language model trained specifically for medical applications. Med-PaLM excels in understanding and generating human-like responses to medical queries, such as providing explanations for complex medical conditions or generating patient summaries. Its training corpus includes a diverse range of medical literature, clinical data, and case reports, making it an effective tool for clinical decision support and medical research. Another notable medical large model **ChatDoctor** [10], which is fine-tuned with real-world patient-doctor interactions, represents a significant advancement in medical LLMs, demonstrating a significant improvement in understanding patient inquiries and providing accurate advice. At the same time, many Chinese medical models fine-tuned on Chinese corpora have also emerged. **HuatuoGPT** [19] is a Chinese medical large model that combines data generated by ChatGPT with responses from real doctors. Its goal is to provide diagnostic capabilities and useful information similar to that of a physician, while maintaining smooth interactions and content richness. On the other hand, **PediatricsGPT** [18] enhances its medical knowledge and dialogue generation capabilities for pediatric tasks by constructing a high-quality PedCorpus dataset and implementing a systematic training process. Both models represent significant advancements in the field of professional medical consultation using Chinese medical large models.

These models are being continuously refined and applied to various aspects of healthcare, from diagnostics and treatment optimization to drug discovery and genetic research. However, their successful deployment depends on overcoming significant challenges, such as ensuring data privacy, improving model interpretability, and addressing issues related to model generalization across diverse patient populations.

2.2   Parameter-Efficient Fine-Tuning

Training large models from scratch is time-consuming and resource-intensive. To address this, various parameter-efficient fine-tuning (PEFT) methods have been proposed to adapt pre-trained models to specific tasks effectively. For instance, Houlsby et al. [4] proposed the **Adapter** method, which adds small adapter modules at each layer of the pre-trained model and fine-tunes only these modules, reducing the number of parameters to be trained. Li and Liang [9] introduced **Prefix-Tuning**, which adds trainable prefix vectors to each layer of the model, freezing the original model's parameters and fine-tuning only the prefixes for efficient adaptation. Hu et al. [5] proposed **Low-Rank Adaptation(LoRA)**, which decomposes the model's weights into low-rank matrices and fine-tunes only these matrices, significantly reducing the number of trainable parameters. Additionally, Liu et al. [14] proposed **P-Tuning**, which uses trainable continuous prompt vectors instead of discrete textual prompts, achieving better task adaptation, while Ben-Zaken et al. [1] introduced **BitFit**, which fine-tunes only the bias parameters of the model, significantly simplifying the parameter update process. These methods effectively reduce training time and resource consumption while maintaining strong performance on specific tasks and therefore widely used.

2.3   Retrieval-Augmented Generation

Retrieval-augmented generation (RAG) is an advanced approach to leverage external knowledge to enhance generative models. In the RAG process, the process typically involves two phases: retrieval and generation. First, the retrieval mechanism identifies relevant documents from a large-scale corpus based on the query. The retrieved information is then fed as context into a language model that generates responses based on the original input and the retrieved knowledge. This technique has been shown to be effective in reducing model hallucination problems and is very effective in areas such as medicine where knowledge is fine-grained.

There has been a lot of research work on RAG. **GraphRAG** [2] leverages a large language model (LLM) to create a graph-based text index in two stages. First, it generates an entity knowledge graph from source documents. Then, it pre-generates community summaries for groups of closely related entities. When given a question, each community summary contributes to generating a partial response, which is subsequently summarized to produce a final answer. **Knowledge Augmented Generation** [11] addresses key limitations of RAG systems, such as weak reasoning relevance and insensitivity to logical nuances, by integrating large language models (LLMs) with knowledge graphs (KGs). Through LLM-friendly knowledge representation, mutual indexing, and hybrid reasoning, KAG achieves significant performance gains in multihop question answering and professional applications **LightRAG** [3] employs a dual-level retrieval system, which enhances the comprehensiveness of information retrieval by facilitating both low-level and high-level knowledge discovery to recover the limitations including reliance on flat data representations and a lack of contextual awareness, often resulting in fragmented answers that fail to capture complex interdependencies.

3   Task Overview

3.1   Benchmark for the Task

To evaluate the diagnostic capabilities of medical large models on real medical records, we launched a benchmark based on real medical records selected from the Chinese Medical Care Repository[1], which was professionally processed and reviewed by medical experts. In order to more comprehensively evaluate the overall capabilities of the model and ensure its generalization, we organized two rounds of competition. In the first round, we provided training sets and test sets; in the second round, we only provided test sets. The data overview of each round is shown in the Table 1. For further details, please refer to [17].

Table 1. The overview of the benchmark.

Round	Training set	Test set	All
1	2591	648	3239
2	–	1000	1000

3.2   Evaluation Metrics

To evaluate the performance of each team's proposed method, we used the F1 score as the main evaluation metric. The F1 score is the harmonic mean of precision and recall, and is a balanced measure of the accuracy of the model by

---

[1] https://www.yiigle.com/Journal/Detail/185.

considering both false positives and false negatives. It is particularly suitable for tasks with class imbalance or where precision and recall are equally important. The final ranking of each team is obtained by averaging the F1 scores of the two round test sets.

The F1 score is calculated as follows:

$$F_1 = 2 \times \frac{\text{Precision} \times \text{Recall}}{\text{Precision} + \text{Recall}}, \tag{1}$$

where precision is defined as the ratio of true positive predictions to the total number of positive predictions, and recall is defined as the ratio of true positive predictions to the total number of actual positive instances:

$$\text{Precision} = \frac{\text{True Positives (TP)}}{\text{TP} + \text{False Positives (FP)}}, \tag{2}$$

$$\text{Recall} = \frac{\text{TP}}{\text{TP} + \text{False Negatives (FN)}}. \tag{3}$$

4   Participating Teams and Methods

4.1   Participating Teams

This shared task is held in CHIP-2024 Conference as Shared Task 3. We held this shared task with the help the Tianchi Team, and all the logistics are handled by the Tianchi platform.[2] Totally, 190 teams participated in this task. And 5 teams winned finally, as shown in Table 2.

Table 2. The winning teams and their Micro-F1 scores.

Rank	Institution	First round	Second round	Avg
1 [12]	Zhengzhou University	0.9941	0.9385	0.9663
2 [7]	Northeastern University	0.9932	0.9356	0.9644
3 [6]	School of Electronic Science and Engineering	0.9937	0.9309	0.9623
4 [13]	Zhengzhou University	0.9905	0.9210	0.9557
5 [20]	Beijing Institute of Technology	0.9932	0.9102	0.9517

4.2   Methods of the Winning Teams

In this subsection, we will analyze the techniques employed by each winning team during the fine-tuning and inference stages. Specifically, we will discuss

---

[2] https://tianchi.aliyun.com/competition/entrance/532278.

the strategies they utilized to adapt their models to the task, including fine-tuning methods and the application of RAG techniques. Fine-tuning approaches varied across teams, with some focusing on parameter-efficient strategies such as LoRA to optimize training on limited task-specific data. Others leveraged RAG frameworks to enhance their models by integrating external knowledge retrieval, enabling more accurate and contextually relevant responses. These methods showcase the diverse approaches to balancing efficiency and performance during model adaptation, highlighting innovative solutions to this tasks.

Fine-Tuning Stage. The winning teams leveraged pre-trained large language models (LLMs) as their backbone for fine-tuning on the medical diagnosis tasks, as shown in Table 3. These models, such as Qwen2.5, Glm-4 and InternLM2.5, were chosen for their exceptional natural language understanding and reasoning capabilities.

Table 3. Pretrained model(s) employed by the winning teams.

Rank	Pretrained model(s)
1	Qwen2.5-7B-Instruct + Qwen2.5-14B-Instruct + Qwen2.5-32B-Instruct
2	Qwen2.5-14B
3	Qwen2.5-7B + Qwen2.5-14B + Internlm2.5-7B
4	Qwen2.5-7BInstruct + InternLM2.5-7B-chat
5	GPT-4o

The top four teams employed LoRA or QLoRA to adapt these models to the specific tasks without the need for extensive computational resources. LoRA works by inserting low-rank adapters into specific layers of the model while freezing the rest, significantly reducing the number of parameters that need to be trained.

The training data available for this task is provided by the specific task itself. The distribution of the training dataset is shown in Table 4. The dataset was carefully curated to ensure diversity and representativeness.

Table 4. The overview of the training dataset.

Round	Single Choice	Multiple Choices	All
1	1895	696	2591
2	–	–	–

Inference Stage. During the inference stage, the winning teams implemented a variety of strategies to enhance the performance and reliability of their models. The first, third and fourth ranked teams utilized a voting mechanism, where predictions from multiple models were aggregated to determine the final output. This approach comprehensively considered the consistency of the answers and reduced the impact of individual model errors, thereby improving the overall accuracy of the predictions. Additionally, the third ranked team applied an Error Correction Mechanism to address and correct inconsistent answers from each model.

Additionally, the second-ranked team applied Zero-Shot-CoT [8] and Self-Consistency CoT [16] method, which involve providing intermediate reasoning steps to guide the model towards the final answer. This method was particularly effective in eliciting complex reasoning abilities from the LLMs and was used in conjunction with zero-shot learning to generate reasoning paths without manual annotation.

Different from the above fine-tuning method, the fifth-ranked team implemented RAG approach, which combines the generative capabilities of LLMs with the retrieval of external knowledge, allowing models to leverage up-to-date, domain-specific information. They implemented hybrid retrieval strategies that integrated traditional keyword-based retrieval methods like BM25 with semantic search techniques, enhancing the system's ability to identify relevant case examples. In addition, they also defined a set of matching rules based on common expressions of diagnostic information, which can extract only valuable text from the retrieved documents, effectively reducing the input length and irrelevant noise, thereby improving the accuracy and efficiency of generation.

5   Conclusion

This article provides an overview of the Typical Case Diagnosis Consistency Evaluation Task at CHIP 2024, which is a task that can comprehensively and objectively evaluate the diagnostic capabilities of large medical models. This shared task has been a huge success, attracting researchers from industry and academia. Next, we analyze the techniques used by the winning teams to fully reveal that different techniques are very effective in improving the performance of large medical models.

References

1. Ben-Zaken, O., et al.: BitFit: simple parameter-efficient fine-tuning for transforming pre-trained models. arXiv preprint arXiv:2106.10199 (2021). https://arxiv.org/abs/2106.10199
2. Edge, D., et al.: From local to global: a graph rag approach to query-focused summarization. arXiv preprint arXiv:2404.16130 (2024)
3. Guo, Z., Xia, L., Yu, Y., Ao, T., Huang, C.: LightRAG: simple and fast retrieval-augmented generation. arXiv preprint arXiv:2410.05779 (2024)

4. Houlsby, N., Giurgiu, A., Jastrzebski, S., Morrone, B., Gelly, S., Shao, W.: Parameter-efficient transfer learning with adapters. In: Proceedings of the 36th International Conference on Machine Learning (2019). https://arxiv.org/abs/1902. 00751
5. Hu, E., Shen, Y., Zhang, Y., Koc, C., Sze, V.: LoRA: low-rank adaptation of large language models. In: Proceedings of the 38th International Conference on Machine Learning (ICML) (2021). https://arxiv.org/abs/2106.09685
6. Huang, W., et al.: Assessing diagnostic consistency in clinical cases: a fine-tuned LLM voting and GPT error correction framework (unpublished)
7. Jia, Z., Liu, J., Liu, C.: Utilizing large language models enhanced by chain-of-thought for the diagnosis of typical medical cases (unpublished)
8. Kojima, T., Gu, S.S., Reid, M., Matsuo, Y., Iwasawa, Y.: Large language models are zero-shot reasoners. Adv. Neural. Inf. Process. Syst. 35, 22199–22213 (2022)
9. Li, X., Liang, P.: Prefix-tuning: optimizing pre-trained language models with prefix vectors. arXiv preprint arXiv:2101.00190 (2021)
10. Li, Y., Li, Z., Zhang, K., Dan, R., Jiang, S., Zhang, Y.: ChatDoctor: a medical chat model fine-tuned on a large language model meta-AI (LLaMA) using medical domain knowledge. Cureus 15(6) (2023)
11. Liang, L., et al.: KAG: boosting LLMs in professional domains via knowledge augmented generation. arXiv preprint arXiv:2409.13731 (2024)
12. Liu, H., Song, J., Kong, L., Li, Y., Zan, H., Zhang, K.: The CHIP 2024 shared task 3: the diagnostic consistency task in typical medical case records (unpublished)
13. Liu, X., et al.: Overview of CHIP 2024 shared task 3: the diagnostic consistency task in typical medical case records (unpublished)
14. Liu, X., Xu, W., Yang, L., Dai, Z., Liu, C.W., Yang, Z.: P-tuning: prompt tuning can be comparable to fine-tuning across scales and tasks. arXiv preprint arXiv:2103.10385 (2021)
15. Singhal, K., et al.: Large language models encode clinical knowledge. arXiv preprint arXiv:2212.13138 (2022)
16. Wang, X., et al.: Self-consistency improves chain of thought reasoning in language models. arXiv preprint arXiv:2203.11171 (2022)
17. Wang, Z., et al.: Benchmark of the typical case diagnosis consistency evaluation task in CHIP2024 (unpublished)
18. Yang, D., et al.: PediatricsGPT: large language models as Chinese medical assistants for pediatric applications. arXiv preprint arXiv:2405.19266 (2024)
19. Zhang, H., et al.: HuatuoGPT, towards taming language model to be a doctor. arXiv preprint arXiv:2305.15075 (2023)
20. Zhang, K., Wang, B., Yuan, C., Feng, C., Shi, G.: Reliable typical case diagnosis via optimized retrieval-augmented generation techniques (unpublished)

The Diagnosis of Typical Medical Cases Through Optimized Fine-Tuning of Large Language Models

Haixin Liu, Jinwang Song, Lulu Kong, Yifan Li, Hongying Zan[✉],
and Kunli Zhang

Zhengzhou University, Zhengzhou, China
{lhxin,jwsong,kll,lyfan}@gs.zzu.edu.cn, {iehyzan,ieklzhang}@zzu.edu.cn

Abstract. Large Language Models (LLMs) have gained widespread attention in both academia and industry due to their exceptional performance in natural language processing (NLP) tasks. While many NLP tasks related to healthcare already have established evaluation benchmarks, there is currently no comprehensive evaluation task or standard for diagnostic consistency based on typical clinical cases. In this paper, we introduce a diagnostic consistency evaluation task based on real-world clinical cases. This task integrates diagnostic information for common diseases and aims to provide a comprehensive and objective assessment of the diagnostic capabilities of medical LLMs by accurately simulating the decision-making process of doctors during disease diagnosis. We fine-tuned a general-purpose LLM using LoRA and QLoRA methods, conducting generative end-to-end evaluations during the training process. Additionally, we enhanced model performance through model ensemble techniques. Our approach achieved the highest ranking in both the preliminary and final rounds of CHIP2024: The Diagnostic Consistency Task in Typical Medical Case Records, validating the effectiveness of our method.

Keywords: Large Language Models · Natural Language Processing · LoRA and QLoRA methods

1 Introduction

In recent years, LLMs have sparked a new wave of research in the field of NLP tasks [1,2], demonstrating capabilities akin to Artificial General Intelligence (AGI) and gaining widespread attention from the industry. Over the past two years, significant progress has been made in the development of large models in China, with particularly notable advancements in medical large models. Amidst the rapid growth of medical large models [3], many medical-related NLP tasks now have established evaluation benchmarks. [4] However, diagnostic consistency tasks based on typical medical records still lack comprehensive evaluation frameworks and standards [5].

© The Author(s), under exclusive license to Springer Nature Singapore Pte Ltd. 2025
Y. Zhang et al. (Eds.): CHIP 2024, CCIS 2458, pp. 166–176, 2025.
https://doi.org/10.1007/978-981-96-4298-4_15

At this year's CHIP conference, a tri-party initiative introduced an evaluation task for diagnostic consistency based on real medical records. This evaluation allows participants to gain deeper insights into the performance of artificial intelligence technologies across various diseases and treatment processes, providing robust data support for future applied research.

Task Highlights:

Authenticity: The medical record information includes standard basic details, chief complaints, present illness history, past medical history, and laboratory and examination results, aligning with real clinical diagnostic practices.

Broad Disease Coverage: The medical records encompass a wide range of common diseases from various medical specialties, enabling a comprehensive assessment of the model's interdisciplinary capabilities in medicine.

In-Depth and Comprehensive Assessment: The test includes both single-choice and multiple-choice questions. The multiple-choice section evaluates key diagnoses as well as associated past diseases and complications, making the task highly detailed and challenging.

In CHIP 2024 Shared Task 3 The Diagnostic Consistency Task in Typical Medical Case Records, we utilized Qwen2.5-7B-Instruct, Qwen2.5-14B-Instruct, Qwen2.5-32B-Instruct, Qwen2.5-32B-Instruct-bnb-4bit and Qwen2.5-32B-Instruct-GPTQ-Int4 as primary models [6]. Instruction fine-tuning was performed on these large models using LoRA and QLoRA methods, with generative end-to-end evaluations conducted during training. Evaluation functions were designed based on task-specific metrics to ensure the best LoRA weights were preserved. In addition, We manually implemented the training loop and used an 8-bit optimizer to further improve training speed and memory usage. We also experimented with GPTQ quantized models and Unsloth framework + bnb quantized models to implement QLoRA fine-tuning. Notably, the Unsloth framework enabled fine-tuning of the Qwen2.5-32B-Instruct-bnb-4bit model on a single consumer-grade 24GB GPU. Finally, we employed a model ensemble approach, using voting integration on the options to achieve the optimal results.

2   Related Work

2.1   Large Language Models

LLMs represent significant advancement in the field of NLP in recent years. The emergence of models such as GPT-4 [7,8], LLaMA [9,10], and PaLM [11,12] marks a new pinnacle in the capabilities of pre-trained language models in understanding, reasoning, and generating language. These models are typically built on deep learning techniques, leveraging neural network architectures, particularly the Transformer [13], for language processing and generation. A defining feature of LLMs is their massive number of parameters, often ranging from hundreds of millions to trillions. This extensive scale enables them to excel in language understanding and generation tasks.

The training process of LLMs is generally based on large-scale text datasets and employs unsupervised learning methods for pre-training [14]. During this phase, the model learns extensive language patterns, syntactic structures, and semantic information, gradually enhancing its ability to comprehend natural language. After pre-training, LLMs can be fine-tuned to adapt to specific tasks such as text generation [15], machine translation, and question-answering systems.

2.2   Tuning on Large Language Models

LLMs typically consist of billions to even trillions of parameters. Training such models from scratch not only demands immense computational resources but also involves lengthy processes with substantial costs. As a result, fine-tuning techniques have become essential tools for enhancing the performance of LLMs in specific tasks or domains. There are two common approaches to fine-tuning LLMs: Full Fine-Tuning (FFT) [16] and Parameter-Efficient Fine-Tuning (PEFT) [17]. Full fine-tuning optimizes task performance by adjusting all model parameters, while parameter-efficient fine-tuning focuses on training only a small subset of parameters. This approach significantly reduces computational requirements while retaining most of the advantages of the pre-trained model.

Methodologically, fine-tuning strategies can be categorized into Supervised Fine-Tuning (SFT) [18], Reinforcement Learning with Human Feedback (RLHF) [19], and Reinforcement Learning with AI Feedback (RLAIF) [20]. Each of these methods has distinct applications and trade-offs, but their common goal remains to enhance model performance on specific tasks while minimizing training costs. Given limited computational resources, PEFT has gradually become a popular choice. PEFT encompasses various efficient fine-tuning methods, such as Prompt Fine-Tuning, Prefix Fine-Tuning, and LoRA, with a particular emphasis on QLoRA. QLoRA enables efficient fine-tuning of models with up to 6.5 billion parameters by quantizing and freezing the weights of large language models while training through LoRA modules. This approach significantly reduces training costs, making it an attractive solution for resource-constrained settings. In this paper, we adopted LoRA and QLoRA methods to fine-tune the Qwen2.5 series models.

2.3   LoRA and QLoRA Methods

LoRA and QLoRA are efficient techniques for fine-tuning large language models, designed to reduce computational costs and improve training efficiency. LoRA [21] works by inserting low-rank adapter into specific layers of the model while freezing the rest of the model's parameters. This approach significantly reduces the number of parameters that need to be trained, maintaining the model's performance and adaptability without requiring substantial computational resources. The key advantages of LoRA include computational efficiency, significant cost reduction while retaining task effectiveness, and scalability across different model sizes and tasks.

QLoRA [22] extends LoRA by integrating quantization techniques with low-rank adapter. By applying low-bit quantization, such as 4-bit quantization, to the weights of pre-trained models, QLoRA significantly reduces memory and computational requirements. The quantized weights are frozen, and only the low-rank adapter are fine-tuned, enabling efficient fine-tuning of large models, including those with 6.5 billion parameters, on resource-constrained hardware. The benefits of QLoRA include its reduced memory footprint and cost efficiency, making it particularly suitable for training large models in resource-limited environments. This makes QLoRA a widely adopted approach for efficient model fine-tuning across various applications.

2.4   Ensemble Learning

Ensemble Learning [23] is a machine learning technique that aims to enhance overall performance by combining the predictions of multiple models. The core idea is to integrate diverse models, leveraging their individual strengths to produce better predictions than any single model alone. This approach improves accuracy and generalization by reducing both bias and variance. Common integrative learning methods include:

Bagging: For example, Random Forest trains multiple decision tree models in parallel. Predictions are aggregated using majority voting (for classification) or averaging (for regression), effectively reducing model variance.

Boosting: For example, Gradient Boosting Decision Trees (GBDT) train multiple weak models sequentially. Each model iteratively improves upon the errors of the previous one, gradually enhancing overall prediction accuracy.

Stacking: Predictions from multiple base models are used as inputs for a new model, which produces the final predictions. This approach is well-suited for combining different types of models to improve performance.

By ensemble learning, the model can better cope with the complexity and variety of the data and is suitable for a variety of tasks such as classification and regression.

3   Method

3.1   LoRA Instruction Fine-Tuning for Large Language Models

We used the LoRA method to perform instruction fine-tuning on large language models. LoRA is an efficient approach for fine-tuning large pre-trained language models, particularly effective in scenarios with limited computational and memory resources. The core idea of LoRA is to approximate weight updates using low-rank matrices, significantly reducing the number of parameters required for fine-tuning and improving training efficiency. LoRA achieves this by introducing a small number of additional parameters for low-rank adaptation. When fine-tuning large models, LoRA requires only minimal memory, making it especially suitable for model fine-tuning under resource-constrained conditions. The overall framework of our study is shown in Fig. 1.

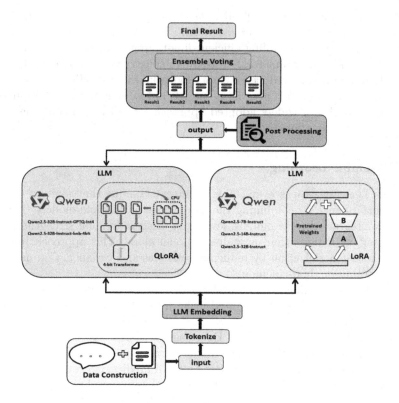

Fig. 1. Overview of model fine-tuning and inference pipeline.

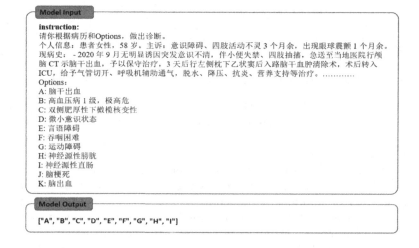

Fig. 2. An illustration of prompt construction.

3.2   Data Processing

We formatted the evaluation task dataset into an instruction-output structure. Since the test set does not include information such as question types (single-choice or multiple-choice), we used only the case descriptions and options from the training data as the context for fine-tuning. This approach ensures consistency in instructions during both training and inference. Additionally, we removed unnecessary spaces in the case descriptions to reduce the input sequence length to some extent. An illustration of prompt template is shown in Fig. 2.

3.3   End-to-End Evaluation in Training

End-to-end evaluation is performed in training by calling model.generate() to preserve the LoRA weights of the best metrics.

3.4   Post Processing

Through post-processing, the model output is converted into the format required for final submission.

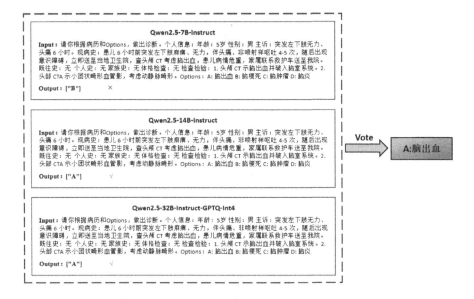

Fig. 3. Single-Choice Voting Mechanism.

3.5   Ensemble Voting

The predictions from a single model often suffer from semantic inaccuracies and short-term memory limitations. To further enhance performance, this study proposes a learning strategy based on a majority voting integration method. By consolidating the outputs of multiple models through voting, the strategy aims to improve accuracy.

For single-choice questions, we applied direct voting integration. For multiple-choice questions, we utilized five models for voting. For each option, we counted the number of times it was selected across the outputs of the five models. An option was included in the final selection if it was chosen by three or more models. Conversely, options selected by fewer than three models were excluded. The final selections comprised all options receiving "three or more votes". The single-choice and multiple-choice voting mechanisms are shown in Fig. 3 and Fig. 4.

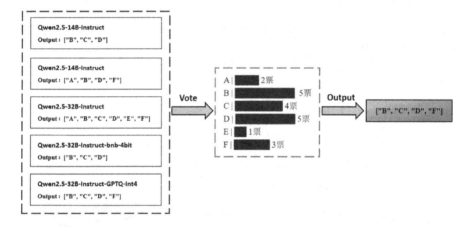

Fig. 4. Multiple-Choice Voting Mechanism.

4   Experiments

4.1   Datasets

The dataset utilized in this study is derived from the CHIP2024 Evaluation Task3, this task is a diagnostic consistency assessment based on a typical medical record, the questions contain single choice and multiple choice questions contestants give the correct option based on the information related to the medical record as well as the options of the question. The total amount of data in the preliminary round is: 3239 data, of which the training set is 2591 and the test set is 648. In order to validate the generalization ability of the model, the organizers conducted a rematch for the teams, with a rematch test set number of 1,000.

4.2   Parameter Settings

During the training process, we used the LoRA framework to partially tune the parameters of the Qwen2.5-32B-Instruct model for 4 epochs of training, and the QLoRA framework to partially tune the parameters of the Qwen2.5-32B-Instruct-GPTQ-Int4 model for 10 epochs of training. We set up end-to-end evaluation in training, every 50 steps, to save the best LoRA weights based on the evaluation results, and we manually stop the training when overfitting occurs, so our epoch settings are relatively large. The learning rate was set to 2e-5 and the batch size was 1. In addition, the parameters used by LoRA in fine-tuning included the LoRA rank of 64, the LoRA alpha of 512, and the LoRA dropout of 0.05. The parameters used by QLoRA in the fine-tuning included the QLoRA rank of 32, the QLoRA alpha of 196, and the QLoRA dropout of 0.05. The parameters of the specific model are listed in Table 1.

Table 1. Experimental parameter settings.

Qwen2.5-32B-Instruct + LoRA	Learning rate	2e−5
	epoch	4
	batch_size	1
	LoRA_rank	64
	QLoRA_alpha	512
	QLoRA_dropout	0.05
Qwen2.5-32B-Instruct-GPTQ-Int4 + QLoRA	Learning rate	2e−5
	epoch	10
	batch_size	1
	LoRA_rank	32
	QLoRA_alpha	196
	QLoRA_dropout	0.05

4.3   Evaluation Metric

The typical diagnosis consistency is evaluated using the classic micro scoring mechanism, including micro Precision, Recall, and F1 scores. In this case, the diagnosis consistency prediction involves predicting the options answer_idx.

When the model's predicted answer_idx overlaps with the ground truth, the number of true positives (TP) is incremented by the quantity of matching options. For example, if the predicted answer_idx is [A, B, D] and the ground truth is [A, B, C], then TP is incremented by 2. If the model predicts options that are not present in the ground truth, the number of false positives (FP) is increased by the count of non-matching options. For example, if the predicted answer_idx is [A, B, D] and the ground truth is [A, B, C], then FP is incremented by 1. If options in the ground truth are not predicted by the model, the number of false negatives (FN) corresponds to the count of unpredicted options.

For example, if the predicted answer_idx is [A, B, D] and the ground truth is [A, B, C], then FN is incremented by 1.

Finally, Precision, Recall, and F1 scores are calculated based on the total TP, FP, and FN across the entire test set.

$$Precision = \frac{TP}{TP + FP} \tag{1}$$

$$Recall = \frac{TP}{TP + FN} \tag{2}$$

$$F1 = 2 \times \frac{Precision \times Recall}{Precision + Recall} \tag{3}$$

4.4 Experimental Setup

The hyperparameters used for the experiment have been written in class Hyper-Parameters. We enabled gradient accumulation and checkpointing to reduce memory usage.

For fine-tuning, we only calculate the cross-entropy loss corresponding to the token in the output part of the instruction.

During evaluation and inference, we uniformly use greedy decoding. The validation set used for evaluation is randomly partitioned from the training set.

4.5 Results and Analysis

Based on running one validation using different models (Qwen2.5-7B-Instruct, Qwen2.5-14B-Instruct, Qwen2.5-32B-Instruct, Qwen2.5-32B-Instruct-GPTQ-Int4) on the training dataset of 2591, the results are shown in Table 2. We observe that Qwen-2.5-32B-Instruct-GPTQ has superior performance. The precision reaches 0.9900, the recall reaches 0.9852, and the F1 score is 0.9883. The experimental results showed that the models with larger parameters were accurate in generating results due to the models with smaller parameters. Finally, we use the ensemble learning method to integrate voting for single and multiple choices to further improve the F1 value. The F1 value reaches 0.9941 on the preliminary test dataset and 0.9385 on the rematch test set, with an average score of 0.9663, ranking first.

Table 2. The results of different models on the dataset.

Model	F1	Precision	Recall	Score
Qwen2.5-7B-Instruct	98.05	98.03	98.10	98.05
Qwen2.5-14B-Instruct	98.38	98.44	97.93	98.38
Qwen2.5-32B-Instruct	98.54	98.70	98.88	98.54
Qwen2.5-32B-Instruct-bnb-4bit	98.78	98.62	98.95	98.78
Qwen2.5-32B-Instruct-GPTQ-Int4	98.83	99.00	98.52	98.83
Ensemble Voting	**99.41**	**99.37**	**99.46**	**99.41**

5   Conclusion

In recent years, LLMs have made significant strides in the field of natural language processing, paving the way for their application in the medical domain. In this paper, we fine-tune large models using the LoRA and QLoRA methods, manually implement the training loop, and employ an 8-bit optimizer to further improve training speed and memory efficiency. Additionally, we incorporate generative end-to-end evaluation during training, setting appropriate evaluation functions based on specific metrics to preserve the best LoRA weights. Finally, we use ensemble methods to enhance model performance. This approach demonstrates the feasibility of applying LLMs to cue learning in medical knowledge quiz scenarios, as well as the effectiveness of integrating ensemble learning with voting mechanisms to improve prediction accuracy. Moving forward, we will continue to focus on fine-tuning the LLMs for a more comprehensive and objective assessment of the diagnostic capabilities of large Chinese medical knowledge models.

References

1. Brown, T.B., et al.: Language models are few-shot learners. arXiv, abs/2005.14165 (2020)
2. Wei, J., et al.: Emergent abilities of large language models. arXiv, abs/2206.07682 (2022)
3. Tian, Y., Gan, R., Song, Y., Zhang, J., Zhang, Y.: ChiMed-GPT: a Chinese medical large language model with full training regime and better alignment to human preferences. arXiv, abs/2311.06025 (2023)
4. Zong, H., et al.: Advancing Chinese biomedical text mining with community challenges. J. Biomed. Inform. **157**, 104716 (2024)
5. Chang, Y., et al.: A survey on evaluation of large language models. ACM Trans. Intell. Syst. Technol. **15**, 1–45 (2023)
6. Bai, J., et al.: Qwen technical report. arXiv abs/2309.16609 (2023)
7. Raunak, V., Sharaf, A., Awadallah, H.H., Menezes, A.: Leveraging GPT-4 for automatic translation post-editing. In: Conference on Empirical Methods in Natural Language Processing (2023)
8. Mao, R., Chen, G., Zhang, X., Guerin, F., Cambria, E.: GPTEval: a survey on assessments of ChatGPT and GPT-4 (2023)
9. Touvron, H., et al.: Llama 2: open foundation and fine-tuned chat models. arXiv abs/2307.09288 (2023)
10. Touvron, H., et al.: LLaMA: open and efficient foundation language models. arXiv, abs/2302.13971 (2023)
11. Bi, B., Li, C., Wu, C., Yan, M., Wang, W.: PALM: pre-training an autoencoding & autoregressive language model for context-conditioned generation. In: Conference on Empirical Methods in Natural Language Processing (2020)
12. Chowdhery, A., et al.: PaLM: scaling language modeling with pathways. arXiv abs/2204.02311 (2022)
13. Vaswani, A., et al.: Attention is all you need. In: Neural Information Processing Systems (2017)
14. Kim, Y., Choi, K.: Entity linking Korean text: an unsupervised learning approach using semantic relations. In: Conference on Computational Natural Language Learning (2015)

15. Radford, A., Narasimhan, K.: Improving Language Understanding by Generative Pre-training (2018)
16. Lv, K., Yang, Y., Liu, T., Gao, Q., Guo, Q., Qiu, X.: Full parameter fine-tuning for large language models with limited resources. In: Annual Meeting of the Association for Computational Linguistics (2023)
17. Hu, Z., et al.: LLM-adapters: an adapter family for parameter-efficient fine-tuning of large language models. arXiv, abs/2304.01933 (2023)
18. Dong, G., et al.: How abilities in large language models are affected by supervised fine-tuning data composition. arXiv, abs/2310.05492 (2023)
19. Zhu, B., Jiao, J., Jordan, M.I.: Principled reinforcement learning with human feedback from pairwise or k-wise comparisons. arXiv, abs/2301.11270 (2023)
20. Lee, H., et al.: RLAIF vs. RLHF: scaling reinforcement learning from human feedback with AI feedback. In: International Conference on Machine Learning (2023)
21. Hu, J.E., et al.: LoRA: low-rank adaptation of large language models. arXiv, abs/2106.09685 (2021)
22. Dettmers, T., Pagnoni, A., Holtzman, A., Zettlemoyer, L.: QLoRA: efficient fine-tuning of quantized LLMs. arXiv, abs/2305.14314 (2023)
23. Kumar, J., Kumar Singh, A., Mohan, A., Buyya, R.: Ensemble learning. Encyclopedia of Biometrics (2019)

Utilizing Large Language Models Enhanced by Chain-of-Thought for the Diagnosis of Typical Medical Cases

Jiqiang Liu[1(✉)] and Chenyang Liu[2]

[1] Faculty of Robot Science and Engineering, Northeastern University,
Shenyang, China
liujiqiang9@qq.com
[2] School of Computer Science and Engineering, Northeastern University,
Shenyang, China

Abstract. In the past two years, the large language model has set off a new wave of research in the field of natural language processing, showing the ability of general-purpose artificial intelligence, which has been widely concerned by the industry. With the rapid development of medical vertical large model, its potential in clinical application has been paid more and more attention. However, there are gaps in the diagnosis of typical medical records. In order to continuously improve the application effect of medical large model in actual clinical scenarios and accelerate the implementation of medical large model, this paper describes the specific situation of our participation in the 10th China Conference on Health Information Processing (CHIP 2024). We used the improved LoRA method for fine tuning, and then used the Chain-of-Thought method for post-processing in the reasoning stage to improve performance. The experimental results show that the F1 score of our method in the final second round of evaluation reaches 0.9356, ranking second, which effectively verifies the generalization and robustness of our method.

Keywords: Large Language Models · Chain-of-Thought · LoRA · Medical Diagnosis

1 Introduction

Artificial intelligence has achieved remarkable progress in the medical field, with applications in medical image analysis, disease prediction, and drug recommendation [3]. These systems have demonstrated their ability to process structured data and provide reliable diagnostic and predictive outcomes. However, significant challenges remain in translating these successes into real-world clinical practice. One of the critical hurdles is diagnostic consistency, which requires aligning AI-generated diagnoses with clinical expert conclusions while effectively handling complex, multidimensional medical data. This includes patient history,

© The Author(s), under exclusive license to Springer Nature Singapore Pte Ltd. 2025
Y. Zhang et al. (Eds.): CHIP 2024, CCIS 2458, pp. 177–190, 2025.
https://doi.org/10.1007/978-981-96-4298-4_16

symptoms, family history, and laboratory results, all significantly influencing diagnostic outcomes. High diagnostic consistency is vital in high-risk areas like oncology and cardiology, where diagnostic accuracy directly impacts treatment efficacy and patient prognosis.

Traditional medical decision models often struggle to synthesize and reason with diverse, unstructured medical data. Large Language Models (LLMs), such as Qwen2.5-14B, offer an innovative solution to these challenges [36]. With their advanced natural language understanding and reasoning capabilities, LLMs can analyze detailed medical records and integrate knowledge from diverse sources, such as medical guidelines and clinical cases, providing valuable decision support to healthcare professionals. These capabilities make LLMs particularly well-suited to tasks requiring deep reasoning and comprehensive data integration, such as ensuring diagnostic consistency.

Motivated by the advantages of LLMs, the China Conference on Health Information Processing (CHIP) 2024 diagnostic consistency evaluation task provides a rigorous platform for testing the capabilities of medical AI models. This task is based on real-world medical records and aims to evaluate the performance of LLMs across various diseases and clinical specialties. This evaluation task has three major characteristics, namely authenticity, wide disease coverage and comprehensive assessment. The dataset mirrors actual clinical practice, encompassing detailed medical records, including patient demographics, chief complaints, present illness history, past medical history, and laboratory test results. Medical cases span multiple departments and common diseases, testing the generalization ability of models across specialties. The task includes single-choice and multiple-choice questions. Single-choice questions focus on the accuracy of primary diagnoses, while multiple-choice questions assess comprehensive diagnostic reasoning, including comorbidities and historical conditions.

To address the challenges presented by this task, we developed a solution that leverages the strengths of LLMs. Our approach utilizes Qwen2.5-14B as the base model and fine-tunes it using the LoRA+. LoRA+ enables us to set different learning rates for the adapter matrices A and B, enhancing feature learning efficiency, allowing the model to better adapt to the nuances of medical data. Furthermore, we iteratively designed and refined prompts to align the model's outputs more closely with the requirements of the evaluation task. To ensure interpretability-a critical requirement for clinical decision support systems (CDSS), we use Zero-Shot-CoT and Self-Consistency Chain-of-Thought methods to implement multi-path reasoning to improve LLMs performance. These tools enable clinicians to understand the rationale behind AI-generated diagnoses, fostering trust and facilitating the adoption of AI technologies in clinical practice. Our results demonstrate that Qwen2.5-14B, when fine-tuned using the LoRA+, delivers consistent and accurate diagnostic outcomes across diverse medical scenarios. By systematically addressing the challenges of diagnostic consistency, this study establishes a robust benchmark for future research and lays the groundwork for broader applications of LLMs in healthcare. In summary, the main contributions of this paper are as follows:

- Prompt Design and Optimization: In diagnostic tasks using typical cases, we design specific prompt templates based on different types of questions to optimize input information and guide the model to generate outputs that meet clinical diagnostic needs.
- LoRA+ Supervised Fine-Tuning: We utilized LoRA+ technology for supervised fine-tuning. LoRA+ improves feature learning efficiency in wide networks by applying different learning rates to adapter matrices A and B, addressing inefficiencies that arise when using a uniform learning rate.
- Inference enhancement: We implement multi-path inference to improve LLMs performance by adopting Zero-Shot-CoT and Self-Consistency chain of thought methods in the inference phase, we improved the model's reasoning ability when processing complex medical records.

2   Related Work

2.1   Large Language Models

In recent years, LLMs have achieved significant advancements in natural language processing, drawing considerable attention from both academia and industry. These models exhibit exceptional language comprehension and generation capabilities through extensive pre-training on vast text corpora [22]. For instance, the GPT series has evolved from GPT-1 to GPT-4, with each iteration increasing in parameter size and enhancing performance. GPT-3 [9] introduced the concept of contextual learning, while GPT-4 [2] made substantial progress in multimodal processing and reasoning abilities. Similarly, the release of the Qwen model series has spurred significant interest within the open-source community, leading to numerous high-quality open-source LLMs developed through instruction fine-tuning or continued pre-training. Inspired by the impressive capabilities of LLMs across various tasks, there has been notable progress in developing large models within the medical domain [32].

LLMs have revitalized various aspects of healthcare delivery. In clinical diagnostics, these models assist healthcare providers by analyzing extensive medical records to identify potential disease indicators, thereby enhancing diagnostic efficiency and accuracy. For example, by integrating patient medical histories, genetic data, and real-time monitoring information, LLMs can generate personalized treatment recommendations [11], advancing the implementation of precision medicine. In medical education, LLMs have become valuable learning tools for both medical students and practitioners, facilitating the mastery of complex medical knowledge through interactive question-and-answer sessions [1]. Additionally, these models have proven beneficial in mental health care, offering psychological counseling and emotional support through natural language generation, thus alleviating the strain on mental health resources [18]. Overall, the applications of LLMs in the medical field underscore their significant potential in addressing various challenges.

2.2 Parameter-Efficient Fine-Tuning

Large Language Models, having undergone extensive pre-training, have acquired general capabilities to address a wide range of tasks. However, researchers have found that the capabilities of LLMs can be further adapted to specific tasks through supervised fine-tuning [16]. Supervised fine-tuning refers to the method of fine-tuning LLMs on natural language instances to equip them with task-specific capabilities. Given the large number of parameters in LLMs, fine-tuning all parameters incurs significant computational costs. This has prompted the development of various parameter-efficient fine-tuning methods, which aim to reduce the number of trainable parameters while maintaining good performance.

Prefix-Tuning [23], introduced by Stanford researchers, adds a series of trainable continuous vectors, called prefixes, before each Transformer layer of a language model. These task-specific prefixes can be considered virtual token embeddings, improving performance across models with varying parameter sizes on natural language understanding tasks. However, the space allocated for the prompt sequence reduces the available space for the input sequence, potentially impacting model performance. In contrast, prompt tuning [21,25] primarily adds trainable prompt tokens to the input layer. Based on discrete prompt methods [19,29], it expands the input text with a set of soft prompt tokens (either in free or prefix form [25]), which are then used to address specific downstream tasks. Microsoft's LoRA [17] introduces low-rank constraints to approximate the update matrix of each layer, thereby reducing the number of trainable parameters for adapting downstream tasks. This allows efficient adaptation to downstream tasks by optimizing the rank-decomposed matrix of dense layers during the adaptation process, while keeping the pre-trained weights unchanged and there is no additional inference delay. LoRA+ [15], an extension of the LoRA framework, enhances feature learning efficiency by applying different learning rates to the adapter matrices A and B, thereby optimizing the learning process.

2.3 Chain-of-Thought

Chain-of-Thought (CoT) [34] is an enhanced prompting strategy designed to improve the performance of LLMs in complex reasoning tasks such as arithmetic reasoning [6,26,27], commonsense reasoning [12,31], and symbolic reasoning [34]. Unlike In-context learning (ICL) [8], which constructs prompts using only input-output pairs, CoT integrates intermediate reasoning steps that lead to the final output into the prompt. Designing effective CoT prompts is critical for eliciting the complex reasoning abilities of LLMs. One approach involves using diverse CoT reasoning paths (i.e., multiple reasoning paths for each question), which significantly boosts performance [24]. Another idea is that prompts containing complex reasoning paths are more likely to activate the model's reasoning abilities, enhancing the accuracy of generating correct answers [10].

However, both approaches require manually annotated CoT, which limits their practical application. To address this limitation, Auto-CoT [35] introduced Zero-Shot-CoT [20], which prompts LLMs to generate CoT reasoning paths without manual annotation. To improve performance, Auto-CoT further clusters the questions in the training set and selects the questions closest to the centroid of each cluster, which better represent the overall training set. While Few-Shot-CoT can be seen as a special prompt case of ICL, the order of demonstrations has a relatively minor impact on performance: in most tasks, reordering examples causes a performance change of less than 2% [34]. Unlike Few-Shot-CoT, Zero-Shot-CoT does not rely on manually annotated task examples. Instead, it directly generates reasoning steps and uses these generated CoT steps to derive the final answer. Zero-Shot-CoT was initially proposed in [20], where LLMs are prompted with "Let's think step by step" to generate reasoning steps and "Therefore, the answer is" to derive the final answer. This strategy was found to significantly improve performance when the model size exceeds a certain threshold, but it is less effective in smaller models, showcasing the emergent abilities of large-scale models. To unlock CoT capabilities for more tasks, Flan-T5 and Flan-PaLM [5] further incorporated CoT into instruction tuning, effectively enhancing zero-shot performance on unseen tasks.

3 Method

3.1 Data Analysis

{
"text" : "个人信息: 患者男性, 35 岁。\n\n主诉: 鼻痒、打喷嚏、流鼻涕、鼻塞 5 天。\n\n现病史: 患者近 3 年来, 进入秋季后均出现鼻痒、打喷嚏、流鼻涕、鼻塞症状, 自行服用感冒药后症状有轻度缓解。\n\n既往史: 无特殊。\n\n个人史: 无特殊。\n\n家族史: 无特殊。\n\n体格检查: 鼻外形正常, 鼻中隔基本居中。鼻甲黏膜颜色苍淡, 呈肿胀状。总鼻道及中下鼻道狭窄, 可见少许渗出物。\n\n检查检验: 血常规示白细胞 10.93×10⁹/L, 淋巴细胞 3.8×10⁹/L, 嗜酸性粒细胞×10⁹/L。",
"diagnosis" : "过敏性鼻炎 (季节性) ",
"id" : "1456643",
"question_type" : "单选题",
"answer" : [" 过敏性鼻炎 (季节性) "],
"options" : {"A": " 急性鼻炎", "B": " 慢性鼻炎", "C": " 过敏性鼻炎 (季节性) ", "D": " 血管运动性鼻炎"},
"answer_idx" : ["C"],
}

Fig. 1. Train data single choice example.

The train data provides a wealth of detailed information, with a specific data sample illustrated in Fig. 1 and Fig. 2, "text" represents the relevant information of the medical record, which primarily includes the patient's basic information, chief complaints, history of present illness, personal history, family history, past medical history, physical examination, and laboratory tests. "Diagnosis" denotes the final diagnostic outcome, "id" serves as the unique identifier for the data, ensuring its uniqueness. "question_type" indicates the type of question, which can be either single-choice or multiple-choice. "options" are the disease choices represented as key-value pairs, formatted as a dictionary. "answer_idx" is the index of the correct answer, with the data format being a list.

Since the problem type is not given in the test set, we need to analyze the training set. In this way, different instruction can be constructed according to

{
"text" : "个人信息: 男性, 66 岁。\n主诉: 间断胸痛 5 年, 加重 1 周。\n现病史: 患者近 5 年间断出现胸骨中下段闷痛不适, 多发于快走时及饱餐后, 休息后可自行缓解。1 周前凌晨睡眠中突发胸痛, 程度较重, 持续 10 分钟后自行缓解。当地医院诊断为 "不稳定型心绞痛", 行冠状动脉造影并植入支架及药物球囊扩张治疗, 术后仍有劳力性胸痛发作, 转至我院拟进一步治疗。\n既往史: 高血压病史 20 年。\n个人史: 长期大量吸烟史。\n家族史: 无特殊家族史。\n体格检查: 血压 153/83 mmHg, 神志清楚, 口唇无紫绀, 颈软, 颈静脉无怒张; 双肺呼吸音清, 未闻及干、湿性啰音, 心界不大, 心率 64 次/min, 律齐, 心脏各瓣膜听诊区未闻及杂音; 腹软, 无压痛、反跳痛, 肝脾肋下未触及, 双下肢无水肿, 双侧足背动脉搏动对称。\n检查检验: 血常规、肝功能、肾功能、血脂、血糖、甲状腺功能、肌钙蛋白 I、肌酸激酶、凝血功能、D-二聚体、尿常规正常范围。心电图示正常范围。超声心动图示左室饱满, 升主动脉增宽 (42mm), 主动脉瓣、二尖瓣、三尖瓣轻度反流, 左室舒张功能减退, 左心室射血分数 56%。颅脑及胸部 CT 未见异常。",
"diagnosis" : "冠状动脉粥样硬化性心脏病不稳定心绞痛; 高血压病",
"id" : "1429570",
"question_type" : "多选题",
"answer" : ["冠状动脉粥样硬化性心脏病不稳定心绞痛", "高血压病"],
"options" : {"A": "冠状动脉粥样硬化性心脏病不稳定心绞痛", "B": "高血压病", "C": "急性心肌梗死", "D": "主动脉夹层", "E": "肺栓塞", "F": "胸膜炎", "G": "肋间神经痛"},
"answer_idx" : ["A", "B"],
}

Fig. 2. Train data multiple choice example.

different topic types. The number of options and question types in the statistical training set are shown in Table 1 and Table 2.

Table 1. Single Choice: The relationship between the type of question and the length and quantity of options.

Length	Quantity
3	1
4	1706
5	120
6	2
7	6

Table 2. Multiple Choice: The relationship between the type of question and the length and quantity of options.

Length	Quantity
7	609
8	34
9	16
10	32
11	4
12	1

It is clearly observed that when the number of options is six or less, it is definitively a single-choice question, whereas when the number of options is eight or more, it is always a multiple-choice question. A special case arises when the number of options is exactly seven, at which time there are only six single-choice questions and 609 multiple-choice questions. Therefore, when the number of options is seven, the probability of it being a multiple-choice question significantly exceeds that of a single-choice question. Consequently, I have enforced a rule where, when the number of options is seven or above, the prompt is set to multiple-choice, and when the number of options is six or below, the prompt is set to single-choice.

3.2   LoRA

In the fine-tuning stage, we utilized LoRA [17] for adaptation, a technique specifically crafted for enabling large language models to acclimate to downstream tasks, known as Parameter-Efficient Fine-Tuning (PEFT). The pivotal idea behind LoRA is to lock the weights of the pre-trained model and infuse trainable low-rank matrices into each layer of the model. This method significantly slashes the number of trainable parameters while still allowing the model to tailor itself to the task in question. In detail, for a fully connected layer within LLMs, where d denotes the input dimension and k the output dimension, LoRA introduces a low-rank decomposition of the weight matrix:

$$W = W_0 + A \cdot B$$

Here,W_0 is the original weight matrix from pre-training, and A and B are the trainable matrices with an adaptive rank r. During fine-tuning, only matrices A and B are subject to updates, while the original weights remain static, thus reducing the trainable parameters from dk to $(d + k)r$.

LoRA provides computational efficiency, memory conservation, and efficient model storage compared to conventional fine-tuning methods, as it obviates the need to store separate copies of the fine-tuned model. Remarkably, despite its parameter efficiency, LoRA delivers performance on a par with or even surpassing full fine-tuning across various natural language processing tasks, positioning it as a promising technology for efficient and effective model adaptation. Despite LoRA's parametric efficiency, it achieves comparable or even better performance than full fine-tuning on a variety of natural language processing tasks, making it a promising efficient and effective model adaptation technique.

It is noteworthy that in LoRA, the learning rates for the adapter matrices A and B are identical. We have enhanced this using the algorithm proposed in [15], where in LoRA+, the learning rate ηA for the adapter matrix A is set to the optimizer's learning rate, and the learning rate ηB for the adapter matrix B is $\lambda * \eta A$, with λ being the value of loraplus_lr_ratio. Specifically, we set the learning rate of matrix B to be a multiple ($\lambda > 1$) of matrix A.

3.3   Chain-of-Thought

Chain of Thought (CoT) is the key to powerful logical reasoning in LLMs. CoT enhances the common sense reasoning ability of large models by requiring the model to explicitly output intermediate reasoning steps before outputting the final answer. This significantly improves the performance of LLMs in complex reasoning tasks. Therefore, we adopt the Zero-Shot-CoT proposed by [20] and simply add "Let's think step by step" at the end of the prompt.

In standard prompt learning, given a question Q, prompt words T, and a parameterized large language model p_{LM}, it is desired to maximize the likelihood of answer A:

$$p(A \mid T, Q) = \prod_{i=1}^{|A|} p_{LM} (a_i \mid T, Q, a_i)$$

Among them, a_i represents the i-th marker.

We use Self-Consistency [33] to enhance the CoT. Specifically, LLMs can use different inference paths when generating the final answer. In multiple inference paths, if the same answer is generated, the answer can be said to be very reliable, that is, correct. On the contrary, if different reasoning paths are used but different answers are obtained, it indicates that the answers generated by LLMs are not very reliable. Given prompt and question, normalize the length of the output, and we weight each inference and answer.

$$P\left(\mathbf{r}_i, \mathbf{a}_i \mid \text{prompt, question}\right) = \exp^{\frac{1}{K} \sum_{k=1}^{K} \log P(t_k \mid \text{prompt, question}, t_1,\ldots,t_{k-1})}$$

Among them, K is the length of the generated token.

$P\left(t_k \mid \text{prompt, question}, t_1, \ldots, t_{k-1}\right)$ is the probability of generating the k-th token (under the $k-1$ constraint), and $P\left(\mathbf{r}_i, \mathbf{a}_i \mid \text{prompt, question}\right)$ is the final weighting coefficient.

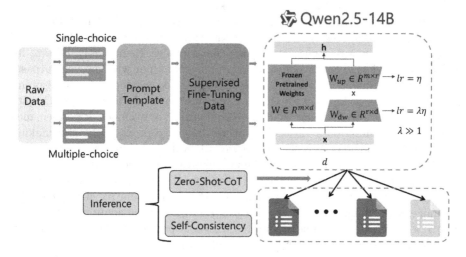

Fig. 3. Overall framework diagram for diagnosing typical medical cases using a Large Language Models enhanced by Chain-of-Thought.

Our overall framework is shown in Fig. 3. We first classify the raw data, construct different prompt words, and then convert case information and diagnostic results into supervised fine-tuning dialogue templates for Lora fine-tuning. We use the Lora+ method to improve feature learning efficiency and model performance, and then use Zero-Shot-CoT and Self-Consistency CoT methods in the inference stage to achieve multi-path inference and improve LLMs performance. Our specific prompt template is shown in Fig. 4.

In general, in diagnostic tasks using typical cases, we design specific prompt templates based on different types of questions to optimize input information and guide the model to generate outputs that meet clinical diagnostic needs.

Prompt Template

你是一个专业的实习医生，我需要你帮医生进行辅助,然后完成单（多）项选择题。
You are a professional intern doctor, and I need you to assist the doctor in completing multiple-choice questions.

医生给出的诊断信息如下：
The diagnostic information provided by the doctor is as follows:

...

你需要一步一步的思考，从医生的诊断信息中逐步分解并锁定关键信息，然后在选项中选择最适合的答案。
You need to think step by step, gradually break down and lock in key information from the doctor's diagnostic information, and then select the most suitable answer from the options.

Fig. 4. Prompt template for diagnosing typical medical cases using Chain-of-Thought.

This process enabled the model to better interpret medical records, identify the primary diagnosis and comorbidities, and make diagnostic decisions more closely aligned with clinical practice. For diagnostic tasks in the medical field, particularly addressing diagnostic consistency across various diseases and departments, we utilized LoRA+ technology for supervised fine-tuning. LoRA+ improves feature learning efficiency in wide networks by applying different learning rates to adapter matrices A and B, addressing inefficiencies that arise when using a uniform learning rate. This fine-tuning significantly enhanced the model's reasoning capabilities in processing typical medical case information, enabling it to deliver more precise and consistent diagnostic outcomes across multiple domains and diseases. We implement multi-path inference to improve LLMs performance by adopting Zero-Shot-CoT and Self-Consistency CoT methods in the inference phase, we improved the model's reasoning ability when processing complex medical records. This approach not only enhanced the model's ability to extract key features from medical records but also enabled it to simulate the clinical reasoning process more accurately, thereby yielding more consistent and accurate diagnostic results.

4   Experiment

4.1   Baseline Models

Given resource constraints, we chose the following model as our baseline.

Glm-4-9b [13]: GLM-4-9B is the open source version of the latest generation of pre-training model GLM-4 series launched by Tsinghua Zhipu AI. In the pre-training stage, a large language model is introduced to participate in data screening, and the understanding and generation ability of the model is significantly improved through 10T of high-quality multi-language data. It also supports long text inference up to 128K context and supports a maximum sequence generation length of 9K.

Qwen2.5-14b [28]: Qwen2.5 is the latest open source large model of Alitong Yiqiwen team, pre-trained on Alibaba's latest super-scale data set, covering up to 18 trillion words, has significantly more knowledge, supports 128K long context, and supports up to 8K long text generation.

InternLM2.5-20B [4]: The Shusheng Puyu series launched by Shanghai Artificial Intelligence Laboratory (Shanghai AI Laboratory) uses a large amount of synthetic data for training, and constantly iterates the model with the help of the model capability flywheel, supporting a maximum of 1024K ultra-long context.

4.2 Experimental Setup

All of our experiments were conducted on a 4 * 3090-24 GB system with Ubuntu 20.04, Python version 3.10, Cuda version 12.1, Pytorch version 2.4.1, and transformers version 4.46. The hyperparameter settings are shown in Table 3:

Table 3. Hyperparameters used in fine-tuning

Parameter	Value
learning rate	1e−4
batch size	1
adam_beta_1	0.9
adam_beta_2	0.95
adam_epsilon	1e−8
weight_decay	0.1
epochs	3
lora_lr_ratio	16
lora_rank	16
lora_alpha	32
lora_dropout_rate	0.05
neftune_noise_alpha	5

4.3 Evaluation Metrics

We used the classic micro scoring mechanism [14], namely Precision, Recall, F1 score. Accuracy refers to the proportion of correctly predicted positive cases, while recall refers to the ability to correctly predict all positive cases Specifically, when the model predicts the number of answer_idx contained in the ground truth, true positive (TP) is added to the corresponding number. For example, if answer_idx is [A, B, D] and the ground truth is [A, B, C], then true positive (TP) is added to 2. If the option answer_idx predicted by the model is not in the ground truth, then false positive (FP) is added to the options that are not in the quantity. For example, if answer_idx is [A, B, D] and ground truth is [A, B, C], then add 1 to false positive (FP). If the options in the ground truth are not predicted by the model, then false negative (FN) is the number that was not predicted, for example: answer_idx is [A, B, D], ground truth is [A, B, C], then false negative (FN) is incremented by 1. Among them

$$P_{\text{micro}} = \frac{\sum_{i-1}^{n} TP_i}{\sum_{i-1}^{n} TP_i + \sum_{i-1}^{n} FP_i}$$

$$R_{\text{micro}} = \frac{\sum_{i-1}^{n} TP_i}{\sum_{i-1}^{n} TP_i + \sum_{i-1}^{n} FN_i}$$

$$F1_{micro} = \frac{2 * P_{micro} * R_{micro}}{P_{micro} + R_{micro}}$$

4.4   Main Results

Table 4. Model performance metrics for different configurations. The best results are highlighted in bold. The second-best result is underlined.

Model	Precision	Recall	F1
GLM-4-9B-base	0.7650	0.7102	0.7366
GLM-4-9B-lora	0.8638	0.8345	0.8489
GLM-4-9B-lora-cot	0.8936	0.9074	0.9004
Qwen2.5-14B-base	0.8245	0.6862	0.7490
Qwen2.5-14B-lora	0.8854	0.8621	0.8736
Qwen2.5-14B-lora-cot	**0.9231**	**0.9240**	**0.9235**
InternLM2.5-20B-base	0.8041	0.6700	0.7309
InternLM2.5-20B-lora	0.8467	0.8127	0.8294
InternLM2.5-20B-lora-cot	0.8845	0.8913	0.8879

Due to the biggest limitation of Self Consistency being time consumption. Therefore, we first not use the self consistency method to all models. The experimental results are shown in Table 4, which compares the results of different models under different methods in Test Set 1. Among them, for the basic ability of the model, Qwen2.5-14B achieved the best performance of 0.7490 based solely on the same prompt words, while InternLM2.5 with a parameter size of 20 B had the worst performance. We speculate that this is due to the adverse effect of synthetic data. The results published in Nature by [30]. indicate that indiscriminate use of model generated content during training can lead to model collapse, which refers to the recursive training of LLMs on data generated in its previous generations over time, resulting in performance degradation. Similarly, [7] have shown in their latest research that even with a small proportion of synthesized data, the model can still stably collapse.

Simple fine-tuning on downstream tasks can significantly improve the model's capabilities, such as Intern LM2.5-20B-Lora increasing 11.88% compared to InternLM2.5-20B-base, Qwen2.5-14B-lora increasing 14.26% compared to Qwen 2.5-14B-base, and GLM-4-9B-lora increasing 13.22% compared to GLM-4-9B-base. However, some of our subsequent CoT and other methods only increased the model's capabilities by an average of about 5.9% based on Lora, such as GLM-4-9B-lora cot increasing 5.71% compared to GLM-4-9B-lora, Qwen2.5-14B-lora cot increasing 5.40% compared to Qwen2.5-14B-lora, and InternL. M2.5-20B lora cot has increased by 6.59% compared to InternLM2.5-20B lora.

Then we adopted the best performing model and method, Qwen2.5-14B-lora-cot, using the Self Consistency method with a reasoning path of 10. Finally, we achieved an F1 score of 0.9356 on the test2, ranking second. This effectively verified the generalization and robustness of our method.

5   Conclusion

This article proposes a method for the consistency task of typical case diagnosis. Firstly, different prompts are constructed for different question types, and then the model is fine tuned using Lora. The Lora+method is effectively used to improve the efficiency of feature learning. Then, in the inference stage, the Self Consistency thinking chain method is used to implement multi-path inference to improve LLMs performance, and Zero Shot CT is further used to improve model performance. Our method achieved a score of 0.9356 in the final test set, jumping from fourth place in the preliminary round to second place in the final, demonstrating the effectiveness of the thought chain paradigm. The paradigm we propose can be easily extended to other natural language processing tasks based on large language models and has good robustness.

References

1. Abd-Alrazaq, A., et al.: Large language models in medical education: opportunities, challenges, and future directions. JMIR Med. Educ. 9(1), e48291 (2023)
2. Achiam, J., et al.: GPT-4 technical report. arXiv preprint arXiv:2303.08774 (2023)
3. Ahmed, Z., Mohamed, K., Zeeshan, S., Dong, X.: Artificial intelligence with multi-functional machine learning platform development for better healthcare and precision medicine. Database 2020, baaa010 (2020)
4. Cai, Z., et al.: Internlm2 technical report (2024)
5. Chung, H.W., et al.: Scaling instruction-finetuned language models. J. Mach. Learn. Res. 25(70), 1–53 (2024)
6. Cobbe, K., et al.: Training verifiers to solve math word problems (2021). arXiv:2110.14168 (2021)
7. Dohmatob, E., Feng, Y., Subramonian, A., Kempe, J.: Strong model collapse. arXiv preprint arXiv:2410.04840 (2024)

8. Dong, Q., et al.: A survey on in-context learning. arXiv preprint arXiv:2301.00234 (2022)
9. Floridi, L., Chiriatti, M.: GPT-3: its nature, scope, limits, and consequences. Mind. Mach. **30**, 681–694 (2020)
10. Fu, Y., Peng, H., Sabharwal, A., Clark, P., Khot, T.: Complexity-based prompting for multi-step reasoning. In: The Eleventh International Conference on Learning Representations (2022)
11. Galitsky, B.A.: LLM-based personalized recommendations in health (2024)
12. Geva, M., Khashabi, D., Segal, E., Khot, T., Roth, D., Berant, J.: Did aristotle use a laptop? A question answering benchmark with implicit reasoning strategies. Trans. Assoc. Comput. Linguist. **9**, 346–361 (2021)
13. GLM, T., et al.: ChatGLM: a family of large language models from GLM-130b to GLM-4 all tools (2024)
14. Harbecke, D., Chen, Y., Hennig, L., Alt, C.: Why only micro-f1? Class weighting of measures for relation classification. arXiv preprint arXiv:2205.09460 (2022)
15. Hayou, S., Ghosh, N., Yu, B.: Lora+: efficient low rank adaptation of large models. arXiv preprint arXiv:2402.12354 (2024)
16. Howard, J., Ruder, S.: Universal language model fine-tuning for text classification. arXiv preprint arXiv:1801.06146 (2018)
17. Hu, E.J., et al.: Lora: low-rank adaptation of large language models. arXiv preprint arXiv:2106.09685 (2021)
18. Hua, Y., et al.: Large language models in mental health care: a scoping review. arXiv, Preprint posted online on January 1, 2024 (2024)
19. Jiang, Z., Xu, F.F., Araki, J., Neubig, G.: How can we know what language models know? Trans. Assoc. Comput. Linguist. **8**, 423–438 (2020)
20. Kojima, T., Gu, S.S., Reid, M., Matsuo, Y., Iwasawa, Y.: Large language models are zero-shot reasoners. Adv. Neural. Inf. Process. Syst. **35**, 22199–22213 (2022)
21. Lester, B., Al-Rfou, R., Constant, N.: The power of scale for parameter-efficient prompt tuning. arXiv preprint arXiv:2104.08691 (2021)
22. Li, J., Tang, T., Zhao, W.X., Nie, J.Y., Wen, J.R.: Pre-trained language models for text generation: a survey. ACM Comput. Surv. **56**(9), 1–39 (2024)
23. Li, X.L., Liang, P.: Prefix-tuning: optimizing continuous prompts for generation. arXiv preprint arXiv:2101.00190 (2021)
24. Li, Y., et al.: On the advance of making language models better reasoners. arXiv preprint arXiv:2206.02336 (2022)
25. Liu, X., et al.: GPT understands, too. AI Open **5**, 208–215 (2024)
26. Miao, S.Y., Liang, C.C., Su, K.Y.: A diverse corpus for evaluating and developing English math word problem solvers. arXiv preprint arXiv:2106.15772 (2021)
27. Patel, A., Bhattamishra, S., Goyal, N.: Are NLP models really able to solve simple math word problems? arXiv preprint arXiv:2103.07191 (2021)
28. Qwen Team: Qwen2.5: A party of foundation models (2024). https://qwenlm.github.io/blog/qwen2.5/
29. Shin, T., Razeghi, Y., Logan, R.L., IV., Wallace, E., Singh, S.: Autoprompt: eliciting knowledge from language models with automatically generated prompts. arXiv preprint arXiv:2010.15980 (2020)
30. Shumailov, I., Shumaylov, Z., Zhao, Y., Papernot, N., Anderson, R., Gal, Y.: AI models collapse when trained on recursively generated data. Nature **631**(8022), 755–759 (2024)
31. Talmor, A., Herzig, J., Lourie, N., Berant, J.: Commonsenseqa: a question answering challenge targeting commonsense knowledge. arXiv preprint arXiv:1811.00937 (2018)

32. Thirunavukarasu, A.J., Ting, D., Elangovan, K., Gutierrez, L., Tan, T.F., Ting, D.: Large language models in medicine. Nat. Med. **29**(8), 1930–1940 (2023)
33. Wang, X., et al.: Self-consistency improves chain of thought reasoning in language models. arXiv preprint arXiv:2203.11171 (2022)
34. Wei, J., et al.: Chain-of-thought prompting elicits reasoning in large language models. Adv. Neural. Inf. Process. Syst. **35**, 24824–24837 (2022)
35. Zhang, Z., Zhang, A., Li, M., Smola, A.: Automatic chain of thought prompting in large language models. arXiv preprint arXiv:2210.03493 (2022)
36. Zong, H., et al.: Advancing Chinese biomedical text mining with community challenges. J. Biomed. Inform. 104716 (2024)

Assessing Diagnostic Consistency in Clinical Cases: A Fine-Tuned LLM Voting and GPT Error Correction Framework

Weikai Huang, Feipeng Dai$^{(\boxtimes)}$, Chengyan Wu, Jiapei Hu, Yifan Lyu, Junxi Liu, and Yun Xue

School of Electronic Science and Engineering (School of Microelectronics), South China Normal University, Foshan 528225, China
{weikaihuang,chengyan.wu}@m.scnu.edu.cn, daifeipeng@126.com

Abstract. Ensuring diagnostic consistency in typical medical cases helps physicians select appropriate treatment plans based on patient records, avoiding discrepancies in treatment strategies caused by differing interpretations among doctors. This consistency ultimately ensures uniformity in medical services provided to patients. This paper proposes a case diagnosis method in the evaluation task of the 10th China Health Information Processing (CHIP 2024). This method fine-tunes and trains three models through the LoRA framework and performs voting. Furthermore, we incorporated a closed-source LLM to refine the results through an error-correction process. Our approach also features post-processing techniques to avoid the need for text alignment. Experimental results demonstrate that the proposed method achieves an accuracy of 0.96, underscoring its effectiveness and reliability.

Keywords: Large Language Models · LoRA Frameworkd · Voting Mechanism · Error Correction Mechanism

1 Introduction

With the rapid development of large language models in the field of natural language, more and more people are paying attention to the capabilities of general artificial intelligence (AGI) demonstrated by the model and applying it to the medical field [1]. Currently, as medical large language models are booming, almost all medical-related NLP tasks have evaluation components, but there is currently no complete evaluation task and standard for the diagnosis consistency based on typical medical records.

The China Health Information Processing is an annual conference organized and conducted by the Medical Health and Bioinformation Processing Professional Committee of the Chinese Society for Information Processing. It is one

W. Huang and C. Wu—Equal contribution.

© The Author(s), under exclusive license to Springer Nature Singapore Pte Ltd. 2025
Y. Zhang et al. (Eds.): CHIP 2024, CCIS 2458, pp. 191–201, 2025.
https://doi.org/10.1007/978-981-96-4298-4_17

of the most important academic conferences in the field of health information processing in China. The 10th China Health Information Processing was themed "Medical Vertical Domain Large Language Model" and organized several evaluation tasks, among which Task 3 focused on the consistency of typical medical record diagnoses. This task integrates diagnostic medical record information of many common diseases, aiming to comprehensively and objectively evaluate the diagnostic ability of the medical large language model by accurately restoring the decision-making process of doctors in diagnosing diseases.

This paper studies the typical medical record dataset provided by the organizer and uses the method of fine-tuning the open-source large language model combined with calling the closed-source large language model API to correct errors to solve the above problems. In terms of model fine-tuning, we used the sft command of the LoRA framework to fine-tune the three models Qwen2.5-7B-Instruct [2], Qwen2.5-14B-Instruct, Internlm2.5-7B-Chat [3]. Among them, the LoRA framework can effectively solve the problem of excessive cost and time caused by fine-tuning the parameters of the entire model, and the use of multiple models for comprehensive voting can reduce the probability of model result errors and improve the stability of the model. When the model voting results are inconsistent, we use the method of calling the closed-source large language model API to correct errors, which can further improve the accuracy of the model. In addition, unlike the common alignment method, we post-processed the data and mapped the content of the model answer to the options, avoiding the confusion and misalignment of the content and options when the model answers. This effectively improves the effect of the model. Our method achieved an accuracy of 0.96 on the test set of this task, proving the effectiveness of the method.

The main contributions of this work are as follows:

- An effective method has been developed to ensure the consistency of typical medical record diagnoses. This paper proposes a method of fine-tuning an open-source large language model combined with a closed-source large language model for error correction, which addresses the problem of poor discrimination of a single model by leveraging the respective advantages of open-source and closed-source models.
- Applying a voting mechanism to the model output. This paper fine-tunes multiple open-source models and votes on them simultaneously. Based on the voting results, it is decided whether to directly output the prediction results or whether further error correction is needed. This method can improve the accuracy of the results.
- A method without aligning answers is applied. We post-process the data so that the output can be directly mapped to the options.

2   Related Work

2.1   Text Classification

Medical text classification has attracted increasing attention in the field of natural language processing. For example, Wang et al. [4]. used CNN networks to solve the problem of automatic clinical text classification. With medical text datasets, researchers can complete disease classification and diagnosis. The main methods include feature extraction, machine learning, and deep learning methods. Early research on text classification mainly relied on manually constructed features and classification using machine learning algorithms. Feature extraction and feature selection are the core of this stage. Common feature representation methods include BOW, N-gram, TF-IDF, word2vec [5], and Glove [6]. Classification algorithms include Naive Bayes, SVM, KNN, and decision tree. Feature selection can select a small number of relevant features from the original features by removing noise, irrelevant, and redundant features [7], but the disadvantage of this method is that the feature representation depends on domain knowledge, has poor scalability, and has limited capture of semantic information and cannot handle complex contextual relationships. With the introduction of deep learning models, text classification has entered a new stage of development. Among traditional deep learning methods, convolutional neural networks (CNN) and recurrent neural networks (RNN) are one of the most representative deep learning models. As a deep learning method, CNN was originally used for computer vision tasks, but in recent years, its application in text classification tasks has achieved remarkable results. The main features of CNN include convolutional layers, pooling layers, and fully connected layers. In text classification, the convolutional layers of CNN are used to extract local features in text, and the pooling layers are used to reduce the dimensionality of features, reduce computational complexity, and enhance the generalization ability of the model. Kim [8] is one of the pioneering works of CNN in text classification applications. He applied CNN to sentence-level text classification tasks, extracted local features in text through a combination of multiple convolutional kernels, and integrated features through pooling layers. As a deep learning model, RNN has a natural advantage in processing sequence data. Unlike traditional models such as convolutional neural networks (CNNs), RNNs can effectively capture temporal relationships and contextual information in texts, so they perform well in text classification tasks. Although RNNs can process time series data, they have the problem of gradient vanishing or exploding when processing long sequences. This makes RNNs perform poorly in processing long texts. To solve this problem, many improved models have emerged. Long Short-Term Memory (LSTM) is a variant of RNN that aims to solve the gradient vanishing problem encountered by traditional RNNs in long sequences. LSTM is widely used in text classification tasks, especially when processing long texts, it has better performance than traditional RNNs. At the same time, because CNNs can extract local features, they are not as effective as RNNs (such as LSTM or GRU [9]) in processing long-range dependencies in texts. Many researchers have tried to combine CNNs with RNNs. For example, Zhou et al. [10] proposed a CNN-RNN hybrid model for long text classification tasks. With the development of large language models, the emergence of BERT [11] has made pre-training and fine-tuning one of the most commonly used methods in NLP tasks. Pre-trained language models learn general language knowledge on a large corpus and then fine-tune it for specific tasks, greatly reducing the task's dependence on labeled data. This method also has good results in downstream tasks [12].

2.2 LoRA Framework

With the development of large language models, more and more researchers are adapting to specific downstream tasks by using fully supervised training and fine-tuning strategies. Fully supervised training refers to training the model using supervised learning on a large dataset, which means that input and corresponding target output are provided for each training sample, and the model learns the mapping relationship between input and output by minimizing the loss function. Fine-tuning refers to further training the pre-trained model on a labeled dataset for a specific task, with the aim of adjusting the model's parameters on a specific task to adapt it to the specific data distribution and objectives of the task. However, how to use lightweight fine-tuning to become a professional model in different fields has become a focus of discussion, and more and more researchers are using lightweight fine-tuning to adapt to different downstream tasks. For this fine-tuning task, we used LoRA technology. LoRA allows us to indirectly train some dense layers in the neural network by optimizing the rank decomposition matrix of the dense layer changes during the adaptation process, while keeping the pre-trained weights unchanged, which significantly reduces the number of parameters compared to full parameter fine-tuning. At the same time, LoRA has the advantages of fewer model layers, easier training, and longer memory time for old knowledge compared to fine-tuning methods such as Adapter Tuning [13], Prefix-Tuning [14], and P-tuning v2 [15]. Therefore, the performance of LoRA is also better than other parameter efficient fine-tuning methods, and is basically the same as or even higher than full parameter fine-tuning.

3 Methodology

3.1 Model Structure

This section introduces the integrated model designed for typical medical record diagnosis consistency problems. The overall structure of the model is shown in Fig 1, which mainly includes three main components: model integration, voting mechanism, and error correction mechanism. In the model integration component, Qwen2.5-7B-Instruct, Qwen2.5-14B-Instruct, and Internlm2.5-7B-Chat are used as basic models. When fine-tuning the model, the sft instruction of the LoRA framework is used for supervised fine-tuning, and batch inference is performed after merging the fine-tuning parameters. For the voting mechanism, each of the three basic models produces a classification result. During the voting process, if multiple wrong answers accumulate and cause the final answer to be wrong, we compare the voting results with a single model, extract the inconsistent options for the single-choice questions, and call the API of the GPT-4 [16] model for error correction. For multiple-choice questions, due to the imbalance of data distribution, the model may make fewer or wrong choices when answering multiple-choice questions. For this, we use the GPT-4 model for error correction for all multiple-choice questions.

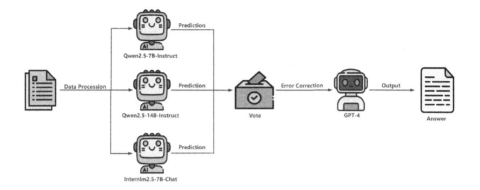

Fig. 1. Model Structure

3.2 Problem Definition

Formally, given an input sentence $s = \{w_1, \ldots, w_L\}$, where w_i represents the i-th token of the sequence, and given the corresponding label set $s = \{l_1, \ldots, l_i\}$, where l_i is the i-th label. The typical case diagnosis consistency task aims to judge and select the correct option mentioned in the sentence based on the medical record-related information and question options in the sentence. The final output $Label = \{w_1, \ldots, w_L\}$, w_i represents the predicted i-th option.

3.3 Data Construction

The training set provided for this typical medical record diagnosis consistency task contains id, text, question_type, opinions, and answer_idx information. The text tag contains relevant information about the medical record, which mainly includes basic information of the patient, chief complaint, current medical history, personal history, family history, past history, physical examination, test examination, etc. Opinions are disease options. Answer_idx are answer options. Due to limited resources, small Chinese models such as ChineseBERT [17] may not be able to solve complex problems with large amounts of text data. Therefore, this experiment uses large language models for reasoning, which usually have strong semantic understanding capabilities. We splice the preprocessed data with appropriate prompts to construct the input of the base model. During the trial, we found that if the large language model directly selects the answer based on the letter options, there will be alignment inconsistencies. Therefore, we let the model directly output the content of the answer through a specific prompt and finally match the content of the letter options output by the model in post-processing to select the final answer.

3.4   Voting Mechanism

Voting mechanisms are often used in text classification tasks in the field of natural language processing to integrate the prediction results of multiple models. For example, Onan et al. [18–20] proposed a weighted voting method for sentiment analysis tasks. This method allows each model to focus on different aspects of the training data, and then combines the output results of each model, so as to effectively solve the text classification task. In the current text classification task, considering that each model has its own advantages and the prediction of a single model may show instability, when the answers output by the three models are consistent, we choose the common answer as the final answer, and when the outputs are inconsistent, the answers of each model are corrected. This method helps to reduce the overfitting of a single model to specific features of the training data, thereby improving classification performance.

3.5   Error Correction Mechanism

When there is a disagreement in the voting results, we will correct the results. We splice the answers output by the model and the new prompt words based on the original constructed data to form a new sentence input into the GPT-4 model for error correction. If it is a single-choice question, the answer of GPT-4 shall prevail. If it is a multiple-choice question, the classification result of the model with the highest accuracy on the validation set shall be used as the benchmark, and based on this, the classification result of GPT-4 shall be combined to check for omissions. This method can reduce the probability of under-selection and omission of multiple-choice questions caused by data imbalance.

4   Experiment

4.1   Data Processing

This dataset comes from the evaluation task 3 of CHIP 2024. The dataset contains 3239 texts related to typical case diagnosis, including basic information, chief complaint, current medical history, past medical history, and question types. The training set contains 2591 texts and the test set contains 648 texts. In the data processing process, this paper adds prompts to each data to help the model make better predictions. The processed data format is shown in Table 1. If it is a direct reasoning case, the prompt output by the model in Table 1 is changed to: "你需要根据病人的病情选择其中符合的病例选项:{predict}"

If the processed data needs to be corrected after reasoning and voting, new prompt words need to be added to the original prompts so that the error correction model can make better inferences based on the previous answers. The data format when calling the error correction mechanism is shown in Table 2.

Table 1. Processed data format for Fine-Tuning

你现在是一名专业的中西医结合的医生，需要为病人进行病例诊断
病人的基本信息和病情如下：**{text}**
给定候选的病例选项有以下：**{options_list}**
你需要根据病人的病情选择其中符合的病例选项内容并输出答案:**{predict}**

Table 2. Processed data format for Error Correction

你现在是一名专业的中西医结合的医生，需要为病人进行病例诊断
病人的基本信息和病情如下：**{text}**
给定候选的病例选项有以下：**{options_list}**
你需要根据病人的病情选择其中符合的病例选项内容并输出答案
下面是先前预测的多选题答案：**{previous_predict}**
请你检查并纠错有误的答案，并按照原始的输出格式输出

4.2 Parameter Setting

In this text classification task, we integrated the three models of Qwen2.5-7B-Instruct, Qwen2.5-14B-Instruct, and Internlm2.5-7B-Chat, and applied the LoRA framework to fine-tune these models. The learning rate was set to 2e-4, the batch size was 8, the epoch was 5, and the deep learning framework used was PyTorch. The parameters of the specific model are shown in Table 3.

Table 3. Model parameters

learning rate	2e-4
batch size	8
epoch	5
LoRA rank	64
LoRA alpha	16
LoRA dropout	0.05
framework	PyTorch

4.3 Evaluation Indicators

This task is scored by the micro mechanism, which includes three scores: Precision, Recall, and F1. The diagnosis consistency prediction includes the prediction option answer_idx. When the answer_idx predicted by the model is included in the ground truth, the true positive (TP) is added to the corresponding number. If the option answer_idx predicted by the model is not in the ground truth, the false positive (FP) is added to the option that is not in the number. If the option in the ground truth is not predicted by the model, the false negative (FN) is the number that is not predicted. Finally, the Precision, Recall, and F1 scores are calculated based on the TP, FP, and FN on the entire test set. These metrics are calculated as follows:

$$Precision = \frac{TP}{TP + FP} \qquad (1)$$

$$Recall = \frac{TP}{TP + FN} \qquad (2)$$

$$F1 = 2 \cdot \frac{Precision \cdot Recall}{Precision + Recall} \qquad (3)$$

The final score can be calculated using these indicators:

$$Score = 0.5 \times (F1 + F1^{'}) \qquad (4)$$

where $F1$ is the score of the first evaluation and $F1^{'}$ is the second evaluation.

4.4   Results

Table 4 shows the performance comparison of our ensemble model after voting, error correction, and data post-processing:

Table 4. Results of the experiment

Model	Method	F1
Qwen2.5-7B-LoRA	Direct predict	0.8068
	With EC	0.8426
	With DP	0.8271
	With EC + DP	0.8531
Qwen2.5-14B-LoRA	Direct predict	0.8695
	With EC	0.8874
	With DP	0.8712
	With EC + DP	0.9047
Internlm2.5-7B-LoRA	Direct predict	0.8011
	With EC	0.8336
	With DP	0.8279
	With EC + DP	0.8465
Qwen2.5-14B-LoRA + Internlm2.5-7B-LoRA	With vote + EC	0.9263
	With vote + DP	0.9204
	With vote + EC + DP	0.9315
Qwen2.5-7B-LoRA + Qwen2.5-14B-LoRA + Internlm2.5-7B-LoRA	With vote + EC	0.9758
	With vote + DP	0.9517
	With vote + EC + DP	**0.9932**

where Direct predict refers to the situation where no data preprocessing and error correction mechanisms are applied, that is, raw data combined with prompts are used for reasoning. And EC stands for error correction and DP stands for data post-processing. F1 represents the score of the first round of testing.

The above data shows that among all the models, Qwen2.5-14B-Instruct has better performance. Additionally, the use of two model integrations can significantly improve the accuracy of the model's answers, and the use of three model integrations can further enhance the model's performance. Furthermore, the error correction mechanism can also enhance the performance of the model. We speculate that the possible reason is that the large language models excel in different directions. Therefore, the method of using large language model integration combined with the voting mechanism can better utilize the advantages of each model and improve performance and robustness. Simultaneously, the error correction mechanism allows the integrated model to utilize closed-source models to check for omissions in the answers, thereby reducing instances where the integrated model makes inference errors when dealing with difficult questions. In addition, data post-processing can also improve the model's reasoning ability to a certain extent, indicating that the method we use to map the answer content to the options can help the model address the alignment problem to some extent.

4.5   Ablation Experiment

To further verify the effectiveness of the error correction mechanism, we conducted an ablation experiment to compare the performance of using only the GPT-4 model for reasoning and using the integrated model combined with the GPT-4 model for reasoning. The experimental results are shown in Table 5:

Table 5. Results of the ablation experiment

Model	Method	F1
GPT-4	Direct predict	0.9461
Ensemble model	With voting + DP	0.9517
Ensemble model	With voting + DP + GPT-4 EC	0.9932

where Direct predict refers to the situation where no data preprocessing and error correction mechanisms are applied, that is, raw data combined with prompts are used for reasoning. And EC stands for error correction and DP stands for data post-processing. F1 represents the score of the first round of testing.

Experimental data show that the integrated model we proposed performs better than the GPT-4 model in evaluating the given dataset, and after combining with the GPT-4 model for error correction, the performance of the integrated model can be significantly improved, proving the effectiveness of the error correction mechanism we use.

5 Conclusion

This paper proposes a new method to address the issue of typical medical record diagnosis consistency. We have innovatively introduced a model integration framework, which comprises three modules: large language model integration, a voting mechanism, and an error correction mechanism. The approach of integrating multiple large language models can leverage the strengths of each model and significantly enhance the model's accuracy for select issues.

References

1. Advancing chinese biomedical text mining with community challenges: J. Biomed. Inform. **157**, 104716 (2024)
2. Binyuan, H., et al.: Qwen2. 5-coder technical report. arXiv preprint arXiv:2409.12186, 2024
3. Zheng, C., et al.: Internlm2 technical report. arXiv preprint arXiv:2403.17297, 2024
4. Yanshan, W., et al.: A clinical text classification paradigm using weak supervision and deep representation. BMC Med. Inform. Decis. Mak. **19**, 1–13 (2019)
5. Mikolov, T., Chen, K., Corrado, G., Dean, J.: Efficient estimation of word representations in vector space. In: International Conference on Learning Representations, 2013
6. Pennington, J., Socher, R., Manning, C.D.: GloVe: global vectors for word representation. In: Alessandro, M., Bo, P., Walter, D. (eds.), Proceedings of the 2014 Conference on Empirical Methods in Natural Language Processing (EMNLP), pp. 1532–1543, Doha, Qatar, October 2014. Association for Computational Linguistics
7. Jianyu, M., Lingfeng, N.: A survey on feature selection. Procedia Comput. Sci. **91**, 919–926 (2016). Promoting Business Analytics and Quantitative Management of Technology: 4th International Conference on Information Technology and Quantitative Management (ITQM 2016)
8. Yoon, K.: Convolutional neural networks for sentence classification. In: Alessandro, M., Bo, P., Walter, D. (eds.) Proceedings of the 2014 Conference on Empirical Methods in Natural Language Processing (EMNLP), pp. 1746–1751, Doha, Qatar, October 2014. Association for Computational Linguistics
9. Chung, J., Gulcehre, C., Cho, K., Bengio, Y.: Empirical evaluation of gated recurrent neural networks on sequence modeling. In: NIPS 2014 Workshop on Deep Learning, December 2014
10. Chunting, Z., Chonglin, S., Zhiyuan, L., Francis, L.: A C-LSTM neural network for text classification. arXiv preprint arXiv:1511.08630, 2015
11. Devlin, J., Chang, M.W., Lee, K., Toutanova, K.: BERT: pre-training of deep bidirectional transformers for language understanding. In: Jill, B., Christy, D., Thamar, S. (eds.), Proceedings of the 2019 Conference of the North American Chapter of the Association for Computational Linguistics: Human Language Technologies, Volume 1 (Long and Short Papers), pp. 4171–4186, Minneapolis, Minnesota, June 2019. Association for Computational Linguistics
12. Zhou, C., et al.: A comprehensive survey on pretrained foundation models: a history from bert to chatgpt. Int. J. Mach. Learn. Cybern. 1–65 (2024)
13. Houlsby, N., et al.: Parameter-efficient transfer learning for NLP. In: Chaudhuri, K., Salakhutdinov, R. (eds.), Proceedings of the 36th International Conference on Machine Learning, volume 97 of Proceedings of Machine Learning Research, pp. 2790–2799. PMLR, 09–15 June 2019

14. Li, X.L., Liang, P.: Prefix-tuning: optimizing continuous prompts for generation. In: Zong, C., Xia, F., Li, W., Navigli, R. (eds.), Proceedings of the 59th Annual Meeting of the Association for Computational Linguistics and the 11th International Joint Conference on Natural Language Processing (Volume 1: Long Papers), pp. 4582–4597, Online, August 2021. Association for Computational Linguistics

15. Liu, X., et al.: P-tuning: prompt tuning can be comparable to fine-tuning across scales and tasks. In: Muresan, S., Nakov, P., Villavicencio, A. (eds.), Proceedings of the 60th Annual Meeting of the Association for Computational Linguistics (Volume 2: Short Papers), pp. 61–68, May 2022

16. Achiam, J., et al.: GPT-4 technical report. arXiv preprint arXiv:2303.08774, 2023

17. Sun, Z., et al.: ChineseBERT: Chinese pretraining enhanced by glyph and Pinyin information. In: Zong, C., Xia, F., Li, W., Navigli, R. (eds.), Proceedings of the 59th Annual Meeting of the Association for Computational Linguistics and the 11th International Joint Conference on Natural Language Processing (Volume 1: Long Papers), pp. 2065–2075, Online, August 2021. Association for Computational Linguistics

18. Onan, A., Korukoğlu, S., Bulut, H.: A multiobjective weighted voting ensemble classifier based on differential evolution algorithm for text sentiment classification. Expert Syst. Appl. **62**, 1–16 (2016)

19. Wu, C., Lin, Z., Fang, W., Huang, Y.: A medical diagnostic assistant based on llm. In: China Health Information Processing Conference, pp. 135–147. Springer, 2023

20. Wu, C., Fang, W., Dai, F., Yin, H.: A model ensemble approach with llm for chinese text classification. In: China Health Information Processing Conference, pp. 214–230. Springer, 2023

Typical Medical Case Diagnosis with Voting and Answer Discrimination Using Fine-Tuned LLM

Xia Liu, Wenhui Fu, Guangyu Zhou, Bohan Yu, Xiaohan Zhao, Yu Song, and Kunli Zhang[✉]

School of Computer Science and Artificial Intelligence, Zhengzhou University, Zhengzhou 450001, China
ieklzhang@zzu.edu.cn

Abstract. The contradiction between the medical services provided by China's healthcare industry and the increasingly growing demand for medical care is becoming more prominent. "AI + healthcare" intelligent diagnosis is an effective way to alleviate this contradiction. Large Language Models (LLMs), with their exceptional natural language understanding and reasoning generation capabilities, have opened new pathways for deeply understanding complex medical texts. However, directly applying LLMs to the medical field may result in hallucinations due to the lack of domain-specific medical knowledge. Additionally, retraining LLMs to update their parameters is not only time-consuming and labor-intensive but also costly. To address this, we adopted the LoRA fine-tuning technique, using Chain-of-Thought (CoT) to design prompt templates for training and inference on Qwen2.5 and InternLM2.5. To further enhance prediction accuracy, we introduced a voting mechanism, selecting the top three models with the highest prediction scores for model fusion. During the post-processing stage, we leveraged the powerful capabilities of LLMs in understanding, generation, and correction to carefully evaluate the top two predictions selected after voting, ultimately determining the best answer option. Experimental results show that our method achieved an F1 score of 99.05% in the preliminary round, with an F1 score of 92.10% in the semi-final, securing the fourth place in the overall ranking, which fully validates the effectiveness of this approach.

Keywords: Intelligent Diagnosis · Large Language Models · Natural Language Processing

1 Introduction

In clinical diagnosis, intelligent diagnosis has become a focal point in the integration of artificial intelligence technology with the medical field. It represents a breakthrough in empowering disease diagnosis and treatment through information technology. This approach holds significant potential for improving the quality and efficiency of diagnosis and treatment, optimizing the allocation of

© The Author(s), under exclusive license to Springer Nature Singapore Pte Ltd. 2025
Y. Zhang et al. (Eds.): CHIP 2024, CCIS 2458, pp. 202–213, 2025.
https://doi.org/10.1007/978-981-96-4298-4_18

regional medical resources, and enhancing public access to healthcare. Consequently, using Natural Language Processing (NLP) technology to process medical record data is an important research pathway for fully exploring the healthcare information embedded within, thereby enabling automated and intelligent disease diagnosis [31].

Early research on intelligent diagnosis can generally be categorized into three main approaches: expert system-based intelligent diagnosis, statistical machine learning-based intelligent diagnosis, and deep learning-based intelligent diagnosis. However, the diagnostic performance of these models is often constrained by the methods of data acquisition or the capabilities of the underlying models. By leveraging the powerful reasoning and generative capabilities of large language models, it is possible to uncover the deep semantic relationships within medical records, further enhancing the performance and accuracy of intelligent diagnostic systems.

In this paper, we utilized LLMs to perform intelligent diagnostic tasks in the medical field. First, we designed prompts for the LLMs based on prompt engineering and CoT reasoning and preprocessed the raw electronic medical record data. Additionally, in the training and inference modules, we fine-tuned the Qwen2.5-7B-Instruct and InternLM2.5-7B-chat models using LoRA, continuously adjusting hyperparameters to experiment and generate the correct options corresponding to patient diagnostic results. To enhance the effectiveness of intelligent diagnosis for this task, we applied model fusion to the top three predictions with the highest scores from the models. Finally, we leveraged the self-correction capability of LLMs to evaluate the answers to multiple-choice questions, producing the final answers. Experimental results demonstrated the effectiveness of this approach, achieving top-five rankings in both the preliminary and final rounds of the competition. Ultimately, our method secured fourth place with a comprehensive F1 score of 95.57%.

2   Related Work

Early intelligent diagnostic research primarily relied on rule-based expert systems and traditional machine learning techniques. While these methods have advanced the development of intelligent diagnosis, they still face limitations in capturing deep features of data. In recent years, deep learning has gained significant attention due to its outstanding performance. With the rapid development of deep learning, research combining deep learning techniques with disease diagnosis has made further breakthroughs. These methods leverage deep neural networks (DNNs), including convolutional neural networks (CNNs) [10,29], recurrent neural networks (RNNs) [11], and generative adversarial networks (GANs) [28], to achieve end-to-end feature extraction and model training. In recent years, with the emergence of pre-trained models, deep learning technology has seen further advancements in the field of intelligent medical diagnosis. Pre-trained models, such as BERT [2] and its variants, have achieved remarkable results in diagnostic applications. Rasmy et al. [15] developed the Med-BERT model by training it on the BERT framework and electronic health record datasets. Experiments conducted on pancreatic cancer and diabetes datasets demonstrated significant improvements in prediction accuracy. Intelligent diagnostic models based on pre-trained models can better capture semantic information from medical literature and clinical records, thereby enhancing the accuracy of disease prediction.

Recently, LLMs have achieved significant breakthroughs in the field of Natural Language Processing. Due to their powerful language understanding and generation capabilities, they have been widely applied to various tasks. In the medical field, LLMs have sparked great interest among researchers in intelligent diagnosis. By leveraging their strong reasoning and generative abilities, applying LLMs to intelligent diagnostic tasks enables a deep analysis of the complex semantic relationships embedded within electronic medical records. Kim et al. [7] used GPT-4 with prompt engineering and discovered that it outperformed mental health professionals in identifying obsessive-compulsive disorder, highlighting the potential of large language models in mental health diagnostics. In contrast to previous studies that employed a single LLM for diagnosis, Wang et al. [19] utilized multiple LLMs, each equipped with specialized medical knowledge, for joint diagnosis. To enhances the accuracy and credibility of the diagnosis, recent studies have incorporated external knowledge into diagnostic tasks, with the external knowledge primarily sourced from corpora [4,12,14,17,18,24–26] in the literature, databases [16,23,27], and knowledge graphs [3,6,21,22,30].

Chain-of-Thought (CoT) reasoning has emerged as a key technique for enhancing the reasoning capabilities of large language models. The central idea of CoT is to explicitly generate intermediate reasoning steps, allowing models to perform complex logical deductions more effectively. Early studies demonstrated that fine-tuning large-scale language models to produce reasoning chains significantly improved their performance on tasks such as mathematical reasoning and commonsense question answering [20]. Moreover, CoT reasoning can also be implemented via few-shot prompting, where a small number of exemplars containing reasoning chains are provided to guide the model in generating similar outputs. Recent advancements have extended the applicability and methodology of CoT. For instance, automated strategies for generating reasoning chains (e.g., Auto-CoT) reduce the reliance on manually crafted exemplars, improving the generalizability of models across diverse tasks. Additionally, some approaches integrate external tools, such as calculators or knowledge bases, to augment the reasoning process, enhancing performance in domain-specific tasks [8].

3   Method

This section introduces the framework designed for the typical case diagnostic consistency task. The overall framework, as shown in Fig. 1, consists of four modules: construction of supervised fine-tuning data, model fine-tuning and inference, model ensemble, and correction of voting results using a large language model.

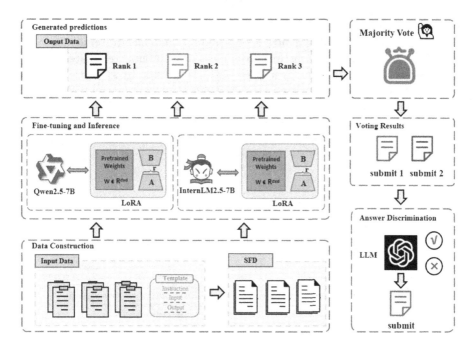

Fig. 1. The overview of our framework.

3.1 Task Description

The "Diagnostic Consistency Task in Typical Medical Case Records" integrates diagnostic medical record information for various common diseases. Its goal is to comprehensively and objectively assess the diagnostic capabilities of medical large language models by accurately simulating doctors' decision-making processes in disease diagnosis. This helps to gain deeper insights into the performance of artificial intelligence technologies across different disease types and various diagnostic and treatment stages. Given medical record-related text, IDs, diagnoses, and options for the questions, the task aims to identify the correct options for each question. The answers may include one or multiple choices.

3.2 Chain-of-Thought Prompting

Prompt Engineering, also known as In-Context Prompting, involves refining prompts through structured text and other methods to guide LLMs in producing desired results. CoT prompting, in particular, enables complex reasoning by incorporating intermediate reasoning steps, facilitating the model's ability to handle more sophisticated tasks. Notably, CoT prompting, a recent approach that leverages step-by-step answer examples to facilitate complex multi-step reasoning, has achieved state-of-the-art performance in arithmetic and symbolic reasoning tasks. Zero-shot CoT [8] is a template-based prompting method designed to enable CoT reasoning without requiring specific examples. It differs from the original CoT prompting [20] as it does not require incremental refinement with small samples, and it is also distinct from most prior prompt templates because it is inherently task-agnostic. By adding "Let's think step by step" to the original prompt, it can elicit multi-step reasoning across a wide range of tasks using a single template. The zero-shot CoT prompting template designed in this paper is illustrated in Fig. 2. Combine the raw electronic medical records (EMRs) provided by this evaluation with the prompt templates designed in this paper to construct the Supervised Fine-tuning Data (SFD).

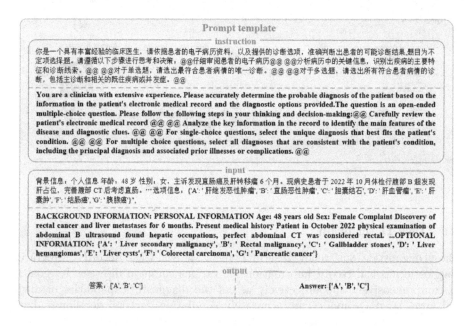

Fig. 2. The zero-shot chain-of-thought prompt.

3.3 Fine-Tuning and Inference

The models selected in this article are Qwen2.5-7B-Instruct [13] and InternLM2.5-7B-chat [1]. The Qwen model is one of the advanced language models that have emerged in recent years. It is based on the Transformer architecture and has acquired extensive linguistic knowledge through large-scale pretraining. Compared to mainstream natural language processing models such as GPT and BERT, Qwen focuses more on applications in generative tasks.

This paper employs LoRA (Low-Rank Adaptation) [5] for efficient fine-tuning in the process of instruction-supervised fine-tuning. This step aims to better adapt the model to the specific medical tasks of this evaluation. The core idea of the LoRA fine-tuning technique is to achieve efficient parameter adaptation by introducing a low-rank decomposition matrix, which is then merged with the pre-trained model weights while keeping the original weights unchanged. This approach enables fine-tuning by adjusting only a few critical parameters, achieving performance that matches or even surpasses full fine-tuning, as shown in Fig. 3. This method significantly reduces memory requirements while ensuring that the trained parameters possess strong representational capabilities.

Denote the pre-training weight matrix as $W_0 \in R^{d \times d}$ and the low-rank matrix as $\Delta W = BA$, with $B \in R^{d \times r}$, with $A \in R^{r \times d}$,where d and r represent the ranks of the pre-trained weight matrix and the low-rank matrices, respectively, with $r \ll d$. Matrices A and B are initialized via random Gaussian distribution and zero initialization, respectively, and contain the trainable parameters (typically derived from the attention layers). During the inference phase, the parameters are used as the merged result of the two matrix components, which is defined as follows:

$$h = W_0 x + \Delta W x \tag{1}$$

The hyperparameter r represents the scale of the trainable parameters, and its specific value needs to be determined based on the size and characteristics of the training dataset. Additionally, ΔW is further scaled by the hyperparameter α, which determines the extent to which the low-rank matrix parameters influence the inference process.

Before training the model, the maximum and minimum token counts across the entire training dataset are detected to select an appropriate value for the cutoff_len parameter, ensuring the model's generalization capability. During training, the dataset is split into a training set and a validation set in an 8:2 ratio. The model parameters are continuously adjusted based on its performance on the validation set. After fine-tuning the model, the question and prompt templates are carefully concatenated to form the input for inference. The fine-tuned Qwen2.5-7B-Instruct and InternLM2.5-7B-Chat models are then used to infer answers to the questions in the test set. Based on the input questions and choices, the model selects the correct answer to the given problems.

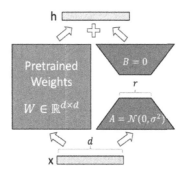

Fig. 3. Schematic Diagram of LoRA Parameter-Efficient Fine-Tuning.

3.4 Majority Vote

Model fusion is a highly significant method in the field of deep learning, aiming to enhance a model's generalization ability, stability, and accuracy by combining the results of multiple models. Among these methods, the voting mechanism is a commonly used approach. Its core idea is to aggregate the predictions of multiple models to achieve better predictive performance. Specifically, the voting mechanism is a strategy based on the principle of majority rule, integrating the predictions of multiple models to improve the model's robustness.

We adjusted the values of the parameters lora_alpha and lora_rank during the fine-tuning process and selected the top three prediction results with the highest scores from the LoRA fine-tuned Qwen2.5-7B-Instruct and InternLM2.5-7B-chat models. These top three prediction results were then merged, and for the single-choice questions, the answers were determined using a majority-vote strategy, where the minority conforms to the majority.

3.5 Answer Discrimination

Leveraging the self-correction capability of LLMs [9], we configured the LLM as a scoring agent to serve as a post-processing module for the entire approach, performing answer discrimination. After the aforementioned voting process, the top two answers with the highest model prediction scores were selected. The GPT-4 was then employed to evaluate these multiple-choice answers. If an answer was correct, it was accepted; if it was incorrect, the GPT-4 corrected it to the right answer. This process was used to generate the final answers for the multiple-choice questions.

4 Experiments

4.1 Datasets and Evaluation Metrics

We conducted experiments using the dataset provided by the CHIP2024 evaluation task for the diagnosis consistency of three typical medical cases. The task provides medical record-related information, including basic demographic information, chief complaints, present illness history, past medical history, and laboratory examinations. The dataset covers multiple departments and a variety of common diseases. The task includes both single-choice and multiple-choice questions, with the latter involving primary diagnoses, related past diseases, and complications, aligning with real-world clinical diagnostic scenarios. This setup allows for a more comprehensive evaluation of the model's multidisciplinary medical diagnostic capabilities. The dataset comprises 3,237 electronic medical records, with 2,590 records in the training set and 647 in the test set. Both the training and test sets include single-choice and multiple-choice questions. The data is labeled with five fields: text, id, question_type, options, and answer_idx. Id: A unique identifier for the data. Text: Medical record information, which mainly includes the patient's basic information, chief complaints, present illness history, personal history, family history, past medical history, physical examination, and laboratory results. Question_type: The type of question, either single-choice or multiple-choice. Options: The disease options, formatted as key-value pairs. Answer_idx: The indices of the correct answers, formatted as a list. During training, the dataset was split into a training set and a validation set at an 8:2 ratio. The specific raw data and its partitioning are detailed in Table 1.

Table 1. The Number of Electronic Medical Records.

Type	The Number of Electronic Medical Records
Train	2072
Val	518
Test	647

The diagnostic consistency task in typical medical case records adopts the classic micro scoring mechanism, including micro Precision, Recall, and F1 scores. The diagnosis consistency prediction involves predicting the answer_idx options. If the number of predicted answer_idx items matches those included in the ground truth, the true positive (TP) is increased by the corresponding count. For example, if answer_idx is [A, B, D] and the ground truth is [A, B, C], the true positive (TP) increases by 2. If the model predicts answer_idx options that are not included in the ground truth, the false positive (FP) is increased by the count of those extra options. For instance, if answer_idx is [A, B, D] and the ground truth is [A, B, C], the false positive (FP) increases by 1. The specific calculation formula is as follows:

$$Micro\,Average\,Precision = \frac{Total\,Number\,of\,Correct\,Answers}{Total\,Number\,of\,Answers\,Recalled\,by\,Model} \quad (2)$$

$$Micro\,Average\,Recall = \frac{Total\,Correct\,Answers}{Total\,Answers\,in\,Test\,Data} \quad (3)$$

$$Micro\,Average\,F1 = \frac{2 \times Micro\,Average\,Precision \times Micro\,Average\,Recall}{Micro\,Average\,Precision + Micro\,Average\,Recall} \quad (4)$$

4.2 Baselines

To validate the effectiveness of our method, we compared it with the following baselines:

LLM-Zero-Shot. For comparison, zero-shot experiments were conducted on the recently released domestic model Qwen72B.

LLM-Fine-tuning Compared to the previous baseline, the Llama Factory framework was used to perform LoRA fine-tuning on the Qwen2.5-7B-Instruct, Qwen2.5-14B-Instruct, and InternLM2.5-7B-Chat models, enabling the generation of multiple-choice answers in the test set.

4.3   Experimental Setup

During training, we used LoRA to fine-tune the parameters of the Qwen2.5-7B-Instruct model. The learning rate was set to 2.0e-5, and the batch size was set to 1. Additionally, the LoRA parameters used for fine-tuning were configured with a lora_rank of 64, a lora_alpha of 128, and a cutoff_len of 2560. The experiments for LoRA fine-tuning of both the Qwen2.5-7B-Instruct and InternLM2.5-7B-Chat models were conducted on a single 24GB NVIDIA RTX 4090 GPU. The specific model parameters are listed in Table 2.

Table 2. Experimental Hyperparameter settings.

Hyperparameter	
learning_rate	2.0e-5
gradient_accumulation_steps	8
lora_rank	64
lora_alpha	128
cutoff_len	2560
lr_scheduler_type	cosine
batch_size	1

4.4   Results and Analysis

We analyze the experimental results of this study, starting with the primary outcomes. Additionally, we conducted ablation studies to evaluate the contribution of each module in the framework.

Main Results. Table 3 presents the overall performance of all baseline methods and our approach on the preliminary test set. Compared to several baseline methods, our approach achieves the highest score with an F1 of 0.9905, demonstrating its effectiveness. When calling the Qwen72B API, the F1 score is only 0.8494. LoRA fine-tuning of the Qwen2.5-7B-Instruct, Qwen2.5-14B-Instruct, and InternLM2.5-7B-chat models yields F1 scores higher than that of LLM-Zero-Shot, indicating significant improvement from fine-tuning. Among them, the Qwen2.5-14B-Instruct model achieves the highest score of 0.9397. Further hyperparameter tuning, by setting the cutoff_len parameter to 2560, results in an F1 score of 0.9701 for the LoRA fine-tuned Qwen2.5-7B-Instruct. This improvement may be due to the fact that when the cutoff_len parameter is set to 1024, some information from the input text is lost, suggesting that the maximum input length of medical electronic health record texts can reach 2560 tokens. In the final round, we tested another test set using our method, achieving an F1 score of 0.9210, which demonstrates the model's good generalization ability.

Table 3. The overall performance of all the compared baselines and our method.

Methods	Models	Score	P	R	F1
LLM-Zero-Shot	Qwen72B	0.8494	0.7831	0.9279	0.8494
LLM-Fine-tuning (cutoff_len=1024)	InternLM2.5-7B-chat	0.9054	0.9002	0.9107	0.9054
	Qwen2.5-7B-Instruct	0.9227	0.8766	0.9739	0.9227
	Qwen2.5-14B-Instruct	0.9397	0.9310	0.9486	0.9397
LLM-Fine-tuning (cutoff_len=2560)	Qwen2.5-7B-Instruct	0.9701	0.9754	0.9648	0.9701
Ours	**Qwen2.5-7B-Instruct**	**0.9905**	**0.9945**	**0.9865**	**0.9905**
w/o Answer Discrimination	Qwen2.5-7B-Instruct	0.9896	0.9918	0.9874	0.9869

Ablation Study. This section presents the results of the ablation experiments. As shown in Table 3, after model ensemble, the F1 score increased from 0.9701 to 0.9896, representing an improvement of 1.95%, demonstrating the effectiveness of the voting method. Removing the LLM-based answer correction module led to a 0.09% decrease in F1, validating the effectiveness of both the voting method and the LLM-based correction module.

5 Conclusion

In this paper, we present the methods used for the CHIP 2024 Task 3 on diagnostic consistency for typical medical cases. We selected the Qwen2.5-7B-Instruct model and employed LoRA fine-tuning, conducting experiments with continuous parameter adjustments to achieve an initial F1 score of 0.9701. Subsequently, we applied model fusion techniques by using a voting mechanism on the top three predictions with the highest scores from the fine-tuned models. For single-choice questions, a majority-voting strategy was adopted. Finally, an open-source LLM was utilized to refine and correct the answers to the multiple-choice questions. The experimental results and analysis demonstrate the effectiveness of the proposed method. In the preliminary round of the evaluation, our approach achieved a final score of 0.9905, ranking fifth. In the final round, it scored 0.9210, ranking fourth, with an overall score of 0.9557, securing fourth place. In the future, we aim to further explore the interpretability of medical LLMs to fully harness the potential of large language models in assisting healthcare professionals in intelligent diagnostic scenarios and other practical applications.

Acknowledgments. This work was supported in part by the Science and Technology Innovation 2030- "New Generation of Artificial Intelligence" Major Project under Grant No.2021ZD0111000, Science and Technology Tackling Project of Henan Provincial Science and Technology Department (232102211039). We would like to thank the anonymous reviewers for their valuable comments and suggestions on the improvement of this paper.

References

1. Cai, Z., et al.: InternLM2 technical report (2024)
2. Devlin, J.: BERT: pre-training of deep bidirectional transformers for language understanding. arXiv preprint arXiv:1810.04805 (2018)
3. Gao, Y., et al.: Large language models and medical knowledge grounding for diagnosis prediction. medRxiv, pp. 2023–11 (2023)
4. Ge, J., et al.: Development of a liver disease-specific large language model chat interface using retrieval augmented generation. Hepatology 10–1097 (2024)
5. Hu, E.J., et al.: Lora: low-rank adaptation of large language models. arXiv preprint arXiv:2106.09685 (2021)
6. Jia, M., Duan, J., Song, Y., Wang, J.: Medikal: integrating knowledge graphs as assistants of LLMs for enhanced clinical diagnosis on EMRs. arXiv preprint arXiv:2406.14326 (2024)
7. Kim, J., et al.: Large language models outperform mental and medical health care professionals in identifying obsessive-compulsive disorder. NPJ Digit. Med. 7(1), 193 (2024)
8. Kojima, T., Gu, S.S., Reid, M., Matsuo, Y., Iwasawa, Y.: Large language models are zero-shot reasoners. Adv. Neural. Inf. Process. Syst. 35, 22199–22213 (2022)
9. Liu, Y., Peng, X., Du, T., Yin, J., Liu, W., Zhang, X.: Era-cot: improving chain-of-thought through entity relationship analysis. arXiv preprint arXiv:2403.06932 (2024)
10. Liu, Y., et al.: A deep learning system for differential diagnosis of skin diseases. Nat. Med. 26(6), 900–908 (2020). https://doi.org/10.1038/s41591-020-0842-3
11. Mei, X., et al.: Interstitial lung disease diagnosis and prognosis using an AI system integrating longitudinal data. Nat. Commun. 14(1), 2272 (2023)
12. Oniani, D., et al.: Enhancing large language models for clinical decision support by incorporating clinical practice guidelines. arXiv preprint arXiv:2401.11120 (2024)
13. Qwen, et al.: Qwen2.5 technical report (2024)
14. Ranjit, M., Ganapathy, G., Manuel, R., Ganu, T.: Retrieval augmented chest X-ray report generation using OpenAI GPT models. In: Machine Learning for Healthcare Conference, pp. 650–666. PMLR (2023)
15. Rasmy, L., Xiang, Y., Xie, Z., Tao, C., Zhi, D.: Med-BERT: pretrained contextualized embeddings on large-scale structured electronic health records for disease prediction. NPJ Digit. Med. 4(1), 86 (2021)
16. Shi, W., Zhuang, Y., Zhu, Y., Iwinski, H., Wattenbarger, M., Wang, M.D.: Retrieval-augmented large language models for adolescent idiopathic scoliosis patients in shared decision-making. In: Proceedings of the 14th ACM International Conference on Bioinformatics, Computational Biology, and Health Informatics, pp. 1–10 (2023)
17. Thompson, W.E., et al.: Large language models with retrieval-augmented generation for zero-shot disease phenotyping. arXiv preprint arXiv:2312.06457 (2023)
18. Upadhyaya, D.P., et al.: A 360° view for large language models: Early detection of amblyopia in children using multi-view eye movement recordings. medRxiv (2024)
19. Wang, H., Zhao, S., Qiang, Z., Xi, N., Qin, B., Liu, T.: Beyond direct diagnosis: LLM-based multi-specialist agent consultation for automatic diagnosis. arXiv preprint arXiv:2401.16107 (2024)
20. Wei, J.: Chain-of-thought prompting elicits reasoning in large language models. Adv. Neural. Inf. Process. Syst. 35, 24824–24837 (2022)

21. Wen, Y., Wang, Z., Sun, J.: Mindmap: knowledge graph prompting sparks graph of thoughts in large language models. arXiv preprint arXiv:2308.09729 (2023)
22. Wu, J., Wu, X., Yang, J.: Guiding clinical reasoning with large language models via knowledge seeds. arXiv preprint arXiv:2403.06609 (2024)
23. Wu, X., et al.: Diagnosis assistant for liver cancer utilizing a large language model with three types of knowledge. arXiv preprint arXiv:2406.18039 (2024)
24. Xia, P., et al.: Rule: reliable multimodal rag for factuality in medical vision language models. In: Proceedings of the 2024 Conference on Empirical Methods in Natural Language Processing, pp. 1081–1093 (2024)
25. Yu, H., Guo, P., Sano, A.: ECG semantic integrator (ESI): a foundation ECG model pretrained with LLM-enhanced cardiological text. arXiv preprint arXiv:2405.19366 (2024)
26. Zhang, H., Li, J., Wang, Y., Songi, Y.: Integrating automated knowledge extraction with large language models for explainable medical decision-making. In: 2023 IEEE International Conference on Bioinformatics and Biomedicine (BIBM), pp. 1710–1717. IEEE (2023)
27. Zhao, W., Deng, Z., Yadav, S., Yu, P.S.: Heterogeneous knowledge grounding for medical question answering with retrieval augmented large language model. In: Companion Proceedings of the ACM on Web Conference 2024, pp. 1590–1594 (2024)
28. Zhou, Q., et al.: A machine and human reader study on AI diagnosis model safety under attacks of adversarial images. Nat. Commun. **12**(1), 7281 (2021)
29. Zhou, S., Huang, X., Liu, N., Zhang, W., Zhang, Y.T., Chung, F.L.: Open-world electrocardiogram classification via domain knowledge-driven contrastive learning. Neural Netw. **179**, 106551 (2024)
30. Zhu, Y., et al.: Emerge: integrating rag for improved multimodal EHR predictive modeling. arXiv preprint arXiv:2406.00036 (2024)
31. Zong, H., et al.: Advancing Chinese biomedical text mining with community challenges. J. Biomed. Inform. 104716 (2024)

Reliable Typical Case Diagnosis via Optimized Retrieval-Augmented Generation Techniques

Kaiyuan Zhang[1], Bo Wang[1], Changsen Yuan[1], Chong Feng[1(✉)], and Ge Shi[2]

[1] Beijing Institute of Technology, Beijing, China
fengchong@bit.edu.cn
[2] Beijing University of Technology, Beijing, China

Abstract. Recent advances in Large Language Models (LLMs) have shown remarkable capabilities in various Natural Language Processing (NLP) tasks. However, their performance in specialized domains, particularly healthcare, is still limited by the lack of domain expertise and output reliability. In this paper, we present a retrieval-augmented framework for the CHIP 2024 Diagnostic Consistency Task in Typical Medical Case Records. Our approach addresses these limitations by combining the generative power of LLMs with the retrieval of relevant medical knowledge. Specifically, we introduce a hybrid retrieval mechanism that integrates traditional BM25 with dense retrieval methods, along with a context compression strategy and self-consistency verification module. This framework enables more reliable and accurate diagnostic predictions by leveraging both contextual similarities and domain-specific knowledge. Our method achieves an average F1 score of 0.9517 on the test set, demonstrating the effectiveness of our approach for specialized medical diagnosis tasks.

Keywords: Case Diagnosis · Large Language Model · Retrieval-Augmented Generation

1 Introduction

Recent advances in Natural Language Processing (NLP) have been driven by the development of Large Language Models (LLMs). Models such as BERT [3], GPT-3 [1], and T5 [14] have demonstrated remarkable generalization abilities across various tasks, including machine translation, question answering, and summarization, due to pre-training on large and diverse corpora. These models leverage billions of parameters, exhibiting an unprecedented capacity to understand, generate, and process human language. Despite their success, LLMs face notable limitations. A major drawback is their reliance on pre-training data. While they can generate coherent output across a wide range of domains, they tend to struggle with tasks requiring domain-specific knowledge. To alleviate this limitation, Retrieval-Augmented Generation (RAG) [8] methods have emerged

© The Author(s), under exclusive license to Springer Nature Singapore Pte Ltd. 2025
Y. Zhang et al. (Eds.): CHIP 2024, CCIS 2458, pp. 214–225, 2025.
https://doi.org/10.1007/978-981-96-4298-4_19

as a promising solution. RAG combines the generative capabilities of LLMs with the retrieval of external knowledge, allowing models to leverage up-to-date, domain-specific information, which enhances their performance on specialized tasks.

The medical domain presents unique challenges which further highlight the limitations of general-purpose LLMs. Medical knowledge is vast and constantly evolving, with frequent updates to diagnostic criteria and treatment protocols. Therefore, medical NLP applications require models capable of processing complex terminology and staying current with developments in the field. Significant progress has been made in applying LLMs to various medical NLP tasks, such as clinical text classification, named entity recognition, and question answering. However, a gap remains in comprehensive evaluation benchmarks for medical diagnostic tasks, particularly those focused on clinical case histories. The China Health Information Processing Conference (CHIP 2024) offers the Diagnostic Consistency Task in Typical Medical Case Records, which evaluates models based on their ability to diagnose diseases from real clinical case data. This task encompasses a wide range of diseases and diagnostic scenarios, including both single-choice and multiple-choice questions, offering a comprehensive evaluation of a model's diagnostic capabilities.

In this paper, we present a novel retrieval-augmented approach for the CHIP 2024 Diagnostic Consistency Task in Typical Medical Case Records. Our method addresses the inherent limitations of LLMs in specialized medical diagnosis by incorporating structured external knowledge and robust verification mechanisms. The key innovation lies in reframing the diagnostic task as a retrieval-augmented generation problem, enabling more reliable and contextualized predictions.

Our framework consists of three main components: (1) a hybrid retrieval pipeline that combines traditional BM25 [16] with dense retrieval methods, (2) a context compression module for efficient information filtering, and (3) a self-consistency [21] verification mechanism for robust diagnosis generation. The hybrid retrieval strategy leverages both lexical and semantic similarities, enhancing the system's ability to identify relevant case examples. The context compression ensures computational efficiency while maintaining essential diagnostic information, while the self-consistency mechanism generates and validates multiple diagnostic hypotheses to improve reliability.

The main contributions of this paper are as follows:

- We employ a retrieval-augmented approach to integrate external knowledge into the large language model, thereby enhancing its performance in specialized domains.
- We employ a hybrid retrieval strategy combining BM25 retrieval and semantic search techniques, thereby enhancing the system's ability to retrieve valuable case information.
- We introduce a post-processing step that includes a context compression module and a self-consistency mechanism, thereby improving the efficiency and accuracy of the system.

2   Related Work

2.1   Text Representation Techniques

Text representation is a fundamental component of NLP, enabling the transformation of unstructured text data into dense vectors. Contextualized word
embedding techniques have been developed to address the limitations of context-
independent embeddings, such as ELMo [12], BERT, and their derivatives. ELMo
employs bidirectional Long Short-Term Memory (LSTM) [4] networks and is
trained on large-scale corpora. It generates embeddings by considering both pre-
ceding and succeeding words in a sentence. BERT builds on the transformer [20]
architecture, leveraging a self-attention mechanism to model bidirectional context effectively. These methods generate word representations dynamically, taking into account the context of each occurrence.

In addition to the representation methods mentioned above, sentence-
level and document-level representations, including Sentence-BERT [15], have
emerged. These transformer-based techniques greatly enhance the performance of knowledge-intensive tasks such as information retrieval by capturing
overall textual meaning. However, these methods focus solely on semantic information, whereas our proposed approach incorporates BM25 retrieval, balancing
semantic understanding with keyword-based information.

2.2   Medical Large Language Models

Pretrained Language Models (PLMs) have significantly impacted Natural Language Processing (NLP). Early PLMs, such as BERT and GPT-2 [13], introduced
innovative techniques such as masked language modeling and autoregressive pre-
training, forming the backbone of the modern NLP paradigm. These models
excelled in task-specific fine-tuning and provided a foundation for subsequent
advances.

The emergence of Large Language Models (LLMs) marked a crucial shift
in the capabilities of language models. LLMs share similar architectures and
pretraining tasks with PLMs but achieve unprecedented performance due to their
substantially increased scale and the resulting emergent abilities [23], such as in-
context learning [1] and reasoning. For instance, T5 reformulated NLP tasks
under a unified text-to-text framework, simplifying fine-tuning across diverse
tasks. GPT-3, with its 175 billion parameters, demonstrated remarkable few-
shot learning capabilities, enabling effective task generalization with minimal
supervision. The evolution continued with GPT-4, which further enhanced its
generative and interpretative abilities, achieving superior fluency and contextual
understanding. These advances highlight the scalability and flexibility of LLMs
in addressing increasingly complex linguistic tasks.

In the medical field, domain-specific LLMs, such as BioGPT [10], Med-
PaLM [19] and Med-Gemini [17], have been developed to address the unique
challenges of biomedical and clinical text processing. These models, trained on
large-scale medical datasets, bridge the gap between general NLP models and

domain-specific medical knowledge, leading to significant improvements in specialized tasks. However, challenges remain, particularly in handling the diversity of medical terminologies and variations in clinical language across different settings. Additionally, ensuring model adaptability to new medical conditions is another significant challenge. In contrast, our proposed approach employs retrieval-augmented generation technique to integrate external knowledge in a non-parametric manner, enhancing the performance of LLMs in specialized domains.

2.3   Retrieval-Augmented Generation Techniques

Retrieval-Augmented Generation (RAG) is an advanced approach that leverages external knowledge to augment generative model. In RAG, the process typically involves two stages: retrieval and generation. First, a retrieval mechanism identifies relevant documents from a large-scale corpus based on a query. Then, the retrieved information is passed into a pre-trained language model, which generates response based on both the original input and retrieved knowledge. This technique has been proven effective in various NLP tasks, such as open-domain question answering, abstractive summarization, and domain-specific applications like medical question answering.

Various methods have contributed to the refinement of this approach. For example, the SKR [22] framework applies retrieval selectively, only when the model lacks the answer, thereby reducing unnecessary retrieval overhead. The GenRead [26] method uses a generative model to generate context and retrieve answers from the produced text. Additionally, iterative methods such as Iter-RetGen [18] integrate the generated information from the prior round, improving retrieval quality through multiple iterations. Frameworks like DSP [7] further enhance the process by decomposing queries into sub-tasks, which can be solved incrementally, making RAG particularly effective for multi-hop reasoning tasks.

As highlighted in recent reviews [28], tasks in the biomedical text mining field, along with their clinical applications, remain challenging. Recent studies have integrated medical Large Language Models (LLMs) with RAG techniques, aiming to address issues like hallucinations and biases. Liévin et al. [9] demonstrate human-level performance on three medical question-answering (QA) datasets by combining chain-of-thought (CoT) reasoning with BM25-based retrieval, utilizing Wikipedia as the external knowledge base. Similarly, Almanac [27], a medical framework based on LLM, leverages an internet browser for dynamic information acquisition and a semantic retriever to extract relevant texts from the database. This approach significantly improves factuality and safety in clinical diagnostics. Furthermore, Self-BioRAG [5] introduces a robust biomedical framework that incorporates a domain-specific instruction-tuned LLM to determine the necessity of retrieval. The framework retrieves relevant texts using the MedCPT [6] retriever and applies a self-reflection mechanism to generate accurate medical explanations and answers.

Additionally, efforts have been made for the benchmark and evaluation of RAG systems in the medical domain. One notable work is Mirage [25], the first comprehensive benchmark for assessing medical RAG systems, including 7663 questions from five medical QA datasets. Furthermore, the study introduces the MedRag toolkit, which integrates domain-specific corpora, retrievers, and LLMs tailored for medical tasks. These works collectively advance the application and evaluation of RAG in healthcare. Our proposed approach optimizes the retrieval and generation process by incorporating a hybrid retrieval strategy and a post-processing step, thereby enhancing the overall performance of the RAG system.

3 Methodology

3.1 Overall Architecture

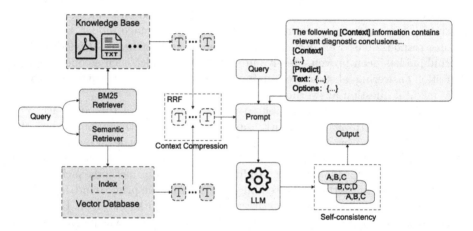

Fig. 1. Overall architecture of our proposed retrieval-augmented framework. Building on pre-constructed knowledge base and vector database, we optimize the retrieval process via a hybrid retrieval strategy and refine the generation process through a post-processing step that include a context compression module and a self-consistency mechanism.

The overall architecture of our method is illustrated in Fig. 1. Specifically, we employ a hybrid retrieval approach that combines a BM25 retriever with a semantic retriever, thereby balancing both contextual and semantic consistency to enhance retrieval performance. Additionally, a post-processing step is performed to compress the retrieved context, and the final results are obtained through a self-consistency mechanism.

To build the medical knowledge base, we crawled case reports from the Chinese Medical Care Repository (2019–2024), a comprehensive database encompassing a wide range of diseases and detailed case information. The raw data, originally in HTML format, was cleaned to extract only the case report sections, removing irrelevant HTML tags and normalizing special characters such as Unicode representations. The resulting knowledge base consists of detailed medical case descriptions, with information pertinent to patient profiles, symptoms, diagnosis and treatment.

On the basis of the knowledge base, we use the BGE [24] model to embed the case reports into dense vectors. These vectors are subsequently indexed and stored in the Chroma vector database, an open-source, high-performance vector database designed for large-scale vector management and retrieval. Chroma employs the Hierarchical Navigable Small World (HNSW) [11] algorithm to construct vector indices, which involves creating multi-layered graphs using node representations of the vectors, thereby enhancing retrieval efficiency.

For each test sample, we use the case information as the query, which is then fed into both the BM25 and semantic retriever. After obtaining the relevant documents, we apply the Reciprocal Rank Fusion (RRF) [2] algorithm to integrate the results. Furthermore, the retrieved information is compressed and used to fill a pre-constructed prompt template, which forms the input to the large language model. Finally, the self-consistency mechanism is applied, performing multiple inferences with the language model to obtain the final diagnostic result.

3.2   Hybrid Retrieval Strategy

The core of the RAG system lies in the retrieval step, where the goal is to acquire the most relevant domain knowledge for a given task. In this work, we employ a hybrid retrieval pipeline that integrates both traditional keyword-based retrieval and semantic retrieval techniques. This hybrid approach significantly enhances the system's ability to retrieve relevant case examples that match the query both in keyword overlap and deeper semantic relationships, thereby improving the accuracy and relevance of the knowledge fed into the subsequent generative model.

Keyword-Based Retrieval. Keyword-based retrieval forms the foundation of many traditional information retrieval systems, which rely on the presence and frequency of query terms within documents to determine relevance. In this approach, a query is typically represented as a set of keywords, and the retrieval process seeks to identify documents containing those keywords, ranked by their frequency.

In this work, we adopt the BM25 retrieval technique, a probabilistic function that ranks documents based on the Term Frequency (TF) and Inverse Document Frequency (IDF). The BM25 formula can be expressed as:

$$Score(Q, d) = \sum_{i}^{n} W_i \cdot R(q_i, d), \tag{1}$$

where Q and d represent the query and the document, respectively. n represents the number of words in query Q, W_i represents the weight of the word q_i, which is its IDF value, and $R(q_i, d)$ denotes the relevance score of the word q_i with respect to the document d. The specific formulas for calculating these two components are as follows:

$$IDF(q_i) = \log \frac{N - df_i + 0.5}{df_i + 0.5}, \tag{2}$$

$$R(q_i, d) = \frac{(k_1 + 1)tf_{td}}{K + tf_{td}}, \tag{3}$$

where N represents the size of the document collection, and df_i denotes the number of documents containing q_i. For a given word q_i, the more documents that contain q_i, the lower its importance and IDF value. tf_{td} represents the term frequency of q_i in document d, k_1 is a tunable parameter, and K is a variable related to document length. When the parameters are fixed, the more frequently q_i appears in document d, the higher the relevance score $R(q_i, d)$.

Semantic Retrieval. Semantic retrieval goes beyond keyword matching by leveraging vector-based representations of text to capture semantic meaning. Instead of relying on exact term matches, semantic retrieval uses pre-trained models to encode both the query and the documents into dense vector embeddings, which are then compared based on their proximity in the embedding space. This approach facilitates the retrieval of semantically relevant documents, making it particularly effective for tasks involving complex or subtle information.

In this work, we use the BGE model, which employs a multi-layer transformer encoder network. Its bi-encoder architecture is shown in Fig. 2. We pre-encode the documents in the knowledge base and store them in the vector database. For each specific query, we embed it and employ an Approximate Nearest Neighbor (ANN) algorithm to retrieve semantically relevant documents from the vector database, using cosine similarity as the metric. The retrieved documents are then ranked based on their proximity to the query vector, and the top-k cases are selected for further processing.

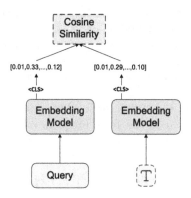

Fig. 2. The bi-encoder architecture of our embedding model. It encodes queries and documents separately and computes their relevance using cosine similarity metric.

3.3   Retrieval-Augmented Generation

After retrieving and integrating relevant documents, we perform context compression to extract the most crucial diagnostic information. This compressed context is then used to fill in a pre-constructed prompt template, which formats the input of the generative model. To further enhance the accuracy of the generated diagnosis, we adopt a self-consistency approach.

Context Compression. Context compression refers to the process of extracting relevant information from a larger body of text, thereby enabling more focused and effective analysis. Unstructured text often contains a large amount of redundant information, with only a small portion being directly relevant to the specific task. Such irrelevant content can hinder task performance. In the medical domain, context compression is particularly critical due to the complexity of clinical cases, which may involve personal details, chief complaints, and test results.

To process the documents, which are characterized by well-defined structural segmentation, we leverage titles as approximate anchors to extract relevant paragraphs. Through a pattern-matching approach implemented with flexible regular expressions, we establish associations between paragraphs and their corresponding titles by identifying structural and semantic alignments. This method enables the selective retention of paragraphs containing key elements related to the title while minimizing extraneous content, and accommodates variations in structure. The process effectively reduces the input length and irrelevant noise, ensuring the inclusion of essential diagnostic information, such as diagnoses, symptoms, and associated clinical observations.

Self-consistency. Self-consistency is a technique used to improve the reliability and robustness of generative models by reducing the impact of model uncertainty or error. It involves generating multiple outputs based on the same input and comparing them to identify the most consistent response. The underlying assumption is that the correct or optimal answer is more likely to emerge when the model consistently generates the same or similar outputs across multiple runs.

In this work, we generate several candidate diagnoses using the same prompt and the final diagnosis is selected based on the most frequent or coherent response. This approach improves the accuracy of the diagnostic process by ensuring that the model's output reflects the most reliable diagnosis. We employ GPT-4o as the generative model.

4   Experiment

4.1   Dataset

The dataset utilized in this work is derived from the CHIP 2024 Evaluation Task 3, which focuses on assessing diagnostic consistency based on real clinical cases. It incorporates diagnostic information covering a wide range of common diseases, enabling a comprehensive evaluation of a medical model's capabilities. In particular, the dataset includes clinical details such as basic patient information, chief complaints, medical history, and diagnostic test results. Additionally, it includes both single-choice and multiple-choice questions, offering a deeper and more challenging assessment of diagnostic accuracy.

The dataset is divided into a training set and a test set, with the former containing 2591 samples and the latter containing 648 samples. Additionally, the second round of the test set includes 1000 samples. The specific test set examples are shown in Table 1. Each sample consists of three fields: id, text, and options, which represent the case ID, the clinical case information, and the candidate diagnoses, respectively.

Table 1. Test set examples containing real clinical cases.

id	text	options
1374591	Personal information: Male, 24 years old. Chief complaint: Headache and dizziness...	A: Malignant syndrome, B: Encephalitis...
1505871	Personal information: Male, 69 years old. Chief complaint: Dyspnea after repeated activities...	A: Heart valve disease, B: Atrial fibrillation...
1366858	Personal information: Female, 11 years old. Chief complaint: Repeated cough for two years...	A: Pneumonia, B: Bronchiectasis...

4.2   Metrics

The task includes three evaluation metrics: precision, recall, and F1 score, with the micro F1 being employed. These metrics are calculated by first determining the true positives (TP), false positives (FP), and false negatives (FN) across all samples in the test set, and then computing the respective values for each metric. The specific formulas are as follows:

$$Precision = \frac{TP}{TP + FP}, \tag{4}$$

$$Recall = \frac{TP}{TP + FN}, \tag{5}$$

$$F1 = 2 \times \frac{Precision \times Recall}{Precision + Recall}. \tag{6}$$

4.3   Results

As shown in Table 2, our full method achieved an F1 score of 0.9932 on the 648 samples in the first test set, with precision and recall values of 0.9955 and 0.9910, respectively. On the 1000 samples in the second test set, the F1 score was 0.9102, resulting in an average F1 score of 0.9517 across two test sets.

Table 2. Experimental results on two test sets.

	Precision	Recall	F1
Test set 1	0.9955	0.9910	0.9932
Test set 2	-	-	0.9102
Avg	-	-	0.9517

To evaluate the effectiveness of our proposed method, we conducted an ablation study on Test set 1, and the results are presented in Table 3. This study consists of three experimental settings:

- Baseline: This approach directly feeds the case information and candidate diagnoses as input into the large language model, which generates the diagnostic results without any enhancement through retrieval or post-processing.
- Our Method (without post-processing): This method employs a hybrid retrieval pipeline to retrieve relevant case information, but does not include context compression or self-consistency checks before performing the diagnosis.
- Our Method (full): This represents the complete RAG framework, which includes both the hybrid retrieval process and the post-processing steps, containing both context compression and self-consistency mechanism, to refine the final diagnostic output.

Table 3. Ablation study results on Test set 1.

Method	Precision	Recall	F1
Baseline	0.9347	0.9203	0.9274
Our Method (-w/o pp)	0.9684	0.9719	0.9701
Our Method (full)	0.9955	0.9910	0.9932

The results indicate that the baseline method, which relies solely on the model's parameterized knowledge, achieved an F1 score of 0.9274. By incorporating the hybrid retrieval pipeline to retrieve relevant case information, both precision and recall saw significant improvements, leading to an F1 score of

0.9701. This demonstrates the effectiveness of our hybrid retrieval strategy. Furthermore, when applying the complete method, which includes context compression and self-consistency checks, all three metrics showed substantial gains, resulting in an F1 score of 0.9932. This further validates the effectiveness of the post-processing steps.

5   Conclusion

This paper proposes a method for the diagnostic consistency task in typical medical case records based on Retrieval-Augmented Generation techniques. Specifically, we employ a hybrid retrieval pipeline that combines traditional keyword-based BM25 retrieval with semantic search techniques, thereby enhancing the system's ability to retrieve valuable case information. Additionally, we introduce a post-processing step that compresses the retrieved context and applies multiple rounds of inference, utilizing the self-consistency mechanism to refine the results. Experimental results demonstrate that our approach significantly improves diagnostic performance, validating its effectiveness.

In the future, we intend to explore the application of the RAG framework to other tasks, particularly within the medical domain. By leveraging effective retrieval strategies and relevant optimizations, we seek to further enhance performance across specific tasks and applications.

References

1. Brown, T.B.: Language models are few-shot learners. arXiv preprint arXiv:2005.14165 (2020)
2. Cormack, G.V., Clarke, C.L., Buettcher, S.: Reciprocal rank fusion outperforms condorcet and individual rank learning methods. In: Proceedings of the 32nd International ACM SIGIR Conference on Research and Development in Information Retrieval, pp. 758–759 (2009)
3. Devlin, J.: BERT: pre-training of deep bidirectional transformers for language understanding. arXiv preprint arXiv:1810.04805 (2018)
4. Hochreiter, S.: Long Short-Term Memory. Neural Computation MIT-Press (1997)
5. Jeong, M., Sohn, J., Sung, M., Kang, J.: Improving medical reasoning through retrieval and self-reflection with retrieval-augmented large language models. Bioinformatics 40(Supplement_1), i119–i129 (2024)
6. Jin, Q., et al.: MEDCPT: contrastive pre-trained transformers with large-scale pubmed search logs for zero-shot biomedical information retrieval. Bioinformatics 39(11), btad651 (2023)
7. Khattab, O., et al.: Demonstrate-search-predict: composing retrieval and language models for knowledge-intensive NLP. arXiv preprint arXiv:2212.14024 (2022)
8. Lewis, P., et al.: Retrieval-augmented generation for knowledge-intensive NLP tasks. Adv. Neural. Inf. Process. Syst. 33, 9459–9474 (2020)
9. Liévin, V., Hother, C.E., Motzfeldt, A.G., Winther, O.: Can large language models reason about medical questions? Patterns 5(3) (2024)
10. Luo, R., et al.: BioGPT: generative pre-trained transformer for biomedical text generation and mining. Briefings Bioinformatics 23(6), bbac409 (2022)

11. Malkov, Y.A., Yashunin, D.A.: Efficient and robust approximate nearest neighbor search using hierarchical navigable small world graphs. IEEE Trans. Pattern Anal. Mach. Intell. **42**(4), 824–836 (2018)
12. Peters, M.E., et al.: Deep contextualized word representations. aabs/1802.05365 (2018). https://api.semanticscholar.org/CorpusID:3626819
13. Radford, A., Wu, J., Child, R., Luan, D., Amodei, D., Sutskever, I., et al.: Language models are unsupervised multitask learners. OpenAI Blog **1**(8), 9 (2019)
14. Raffel, C., et al.: Exploring the limits of transfer learning with a unified text-to-text transformer. J. Mach. Learn. Res. **21**(140), 1–67 (2020)
15. Reimers, N.: Sentence-BERT: sentence embeddings using Siamese BERT-networks. arXiv preprint arXiv:1908.10084 (2019)
16. Robertson, S., Zaragoza, H., et al.: The probabilistic relevance framework: BM25 and beyond. Found. Trends® Inf. Retrieval **3**(4), 333–389 (2009)
17. Saab, K., et al.: Capabilities of Gemini models in medicine. arXiv preprint arXiv:2404.18416 (2024)
18. Shao, Z., Gong, Y., Shen, Y., Huang, M., Duan, N., Chen, W.: Enhancing retrieval-augmented large language models with iterative retrieval-generation synergy. arXiv preprint arXiv:2305.15294 (2023)
19. Singhal, K., et al.: Towards expert-level medical question answering with large language models. arXiv preprint arXiv:2305.09617 (2023)
20. Vaswani, A.: Attention is all you need. In: Advances in Neural Information Processing Systems (2017)
21. Wang, X., et al.: Self-consistency improves chain of thought reasoning in language models. arXiv preprint arXiv:2203.11171 (2022)
22. Wang, Y., Li, P., Sun, M., Liu, Y.: Self-knowledge guided retrieval augmentation for large language models. arXiv preprint arXiv:2310.05002 (2023)
23. Wei, J., et al.: Emergent abilities of large language models. arXiv preprint arXiv:2206.07682 (2022)
24. Xiao, S., Liu, Z., Zhang, P., Muennighof, N.: C-pack: packaged resources to advance general Chinese embedding. arXiv preprint arXiv:2309.07597 (2023)
25. Xiong, G., Jin, Q., Lu, Z., Zhang, A.: Benchmarking retrieval-augmented generation for medicine. arXiv preprint arXiv:2402.13178 (2024)
26. Yu, W., et al.: Generate rather than retrieve: large language models are strong context generators. arXiv preprint arXiv:2209.10063 (2022)
27. Zakka, C., et al.: Almanac-retrieval-augmented language models for clinical medicine. NEJM AI **1**(2), AIoa2300068 (2024)
28. Zong, H., et al.: Advancing Chinese biomedical text mining with community challenges. J. Biomed. Inform. 104716 (2024)

Author Index

© The Editor(s) (if applicable) and The Author(s), under exclusive license
to Springer Nature Singapore Pte Ltd. 2025
Y. Zhang et al. (Eds.): CHIP 2024, CCIS 2458, pp. 227–228, 2025.
https://doi.org/10.1007/978-981-96-4298-4

Printed in the United States
by Baker & Taylor Publisher Services